Men's Health
HANDBOOK

Men's Health
HANDBOOK

Practical Advice on Exercise, Sex, Nutrition, Stress Control, Disease Prevention, Age Reversal and More

By the Editors of
Men's Health Magazine

Rodale Press, Emmaus, Pennsylvania

"Female Sex Secrets" excerpted from *Love Lessons* by Curtis Pesman. Copyright © 1992 by Curtis Pesman. Reprinted by permission of Sterling Lord Literistic, Inc.

Library of Congress Cataloging-in-Publication Data

Men's health handbook : practical advice on exercise, sex, nutrition,
   stress control, disease prevention, age reversal and more / by the
   editors of men's health magazine.
      p. cm.
   Includes index.
   ISBN 0–87596–226–2 hardcover
   1. Men—Health and hygiene. 2. Men—Mental health. I. Men's
health (Magazine)
  RA777.8.M465 1994
613′. 04234—dc20   94–6942
                                                  CIP

Distributed in the book trade by St. Martin's Press

2 4 6 8 10 9 7 5 3 1 hardcover

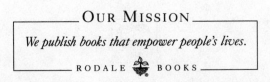

OUR MISSION

We publish books that empower people's lives.

RODALE ✿ BOOKS

Men's Health Handbook Staff

EXECUTIVE EDITOR, *Men's Health* Magazine: Michael Lafavore
EDITOR, *Prevention* Magazine: Mark Bricklin
SENIOR MANAGING EDITOR: Patricia Fisher
SENIOR EDITOR: Russell Wild
COVER AND BOOK DESIGNER: Acey Lee
BOOK LAYOUT: Ayers/Johanek Publication Design
PROJECT COORDINATOR: Roberta Mulliner
COPY EDITOR: Durrae Johanek
MANAGING EDITOR, *Men's Health* Magazine: Steven Slon
RESEARCH EDITOR, *Men's Health* Magazine: Melissa Gotthardt
OFFICE STAFF: Julie Kehs, Mary Lou Stephen
OFFICE MANAGER, *Men's Health* Magazine: Susan Campbell

PREVENTION MAGAZINE HEALTH BOOKS
EDITOR-IN-CHIEF, Rodale Books: Bill Gottlieb
EXECUTIVE EDITOR: Debora A. Tkac
ART DIRECTOR: Jane Colby Knutila
RESEARCH MANAGER: Ann Gossy Yermish

NOTICE

This book is intended as a reference volume only, not as a medical manual. The information given here is designed to help you make informed decisions about your health. It is not intended as a substitute for any treatment that may have been prescribed by your doctor. If you suspect that you have a medical problem, we urge you to seek competent medical help.

Contents

1 HOW A MAN STAYS YOUNG

Want to stay younger longer? Here's the *Men's Health* Look-Good, Feel-Great, Head-to-Toe, Anti-Aging Plan to tell you how to do it.

With the right kind of upkeep, your body can be as tough at 50 as it was at 20—maybe tougher. The secret is training smart.

It's not what you've got; it's how you use it. Here's a guide to maximizing your brain power—at any age.

There's nothing more empowering for a man than to meet his fears and overcome them. So take some risks now and then. The doctor says it will be good for you.

2 HEALTHY EATS

4 MAN-TO-MAN TALK

5 THE WOMEN IN OUR LIVES

6 SEX

7 DISEASE-FREE LIVING

9   BOD LIKE A ROCK

10 TAKING CARE OF BUSINESS

11 ASK *MEN'S HEALTH*

PART 1

How a Man Stays Young

Long-Distance Youth

Want to stay younger longer? Here's the *Men's Health* Look-Good, Feel-Great, Head-to-Toe, Anti-Aging Plan to tell you how to do it.

Aging has a way of leapfrogging up your list of concerns—from somewhere below "I'd better clean out those rain gutters soon" to "Alert! Alert! Top Priority! Code Red!"—in short order. The catalyst might be noticing a wrinkle that wasn't there the last time you looked, trying on a favorite shirt that's suddenly become too tight or playing a routine game of tennis and finding yourself creaky and sore afterward. One day you're thinking of yourself as a young man; the next day you're not so sure.

Fortunately, doctors and researchers are starting to pay as much attention to the subject of aging as the rest of us are. They're working to better understand the changes that come as we get older and what can be done about them. One thing is already clear from their studies: Aging is inevitable—there's no way to stop the clock—but a gradual decline in good health and good looks isn't.

"Many of the things we blame on aging really have nothing to do with getting older," says Ben Douglas, Ph.D., professor of anatomy at the University of Mississippi Medical Center and author of *AgeLess: Living Younger Longer.* He and others believe that we're genetically programmed to age at a certain rate but that most people are sapped of an extra measure of youth by diseases and a gradual buildup of preventable niggling insults to the body. As a rule, experts say, people could look younger, feel more vital and live much longer than they do.

"People should be concerned about aging from the earliest stages of their lives," says Huber Warner, Ph.D., of the National Institute on Aging (NIA). "The problems that lead to aging are cumulative, and the sooner you start correcting them, the better off you are in the long run. I've lived by that advice myself, and at age 55, my own experience tells me I feel better for it."

How can we stay young longer? *Men's Health* called on a wide-ranging field of experts on aging and the problems that attend it and asked them that question. This is the best of their advice.

Get Pumping

A regular weight-training plan can make you feel—and look—decades younger. Research indicates that building muscle strength provides greater benefits to your health and vitality than previously thought. Combined with a regimen of aerobic exercise, it strengthens your heart, boosts energy levels and protects you from injuries. It'll even improve your sex life, says Mark H. Cline, Ph.D., of the Male Health Center in Dallas. "When you're physically stronger, you're more robust, you have more energy and you're more likely to be sexually active."

Plus, it helps keep you looking great. Weight training shapes and tones muscles better than aerobic conditioning, and it wards off flab. "As a result, the average man who lifts weights will look even better than an endurance athlete when they're both older," says John Holloszy, M.D., a researcher at Washington University School of Medicine in St. Louis.

It's never too late to take up weight training. According to Tufts University researchers, even people in their nineties were able to increase their leg strength by as much as 200 percent by working out on weight-training equipment. It only takes one weight workout per week to maintain strength well into old age, once you've made your initial gains (which takes about ten weeks of lifting two or three times a week).

Take Aspirin

Nothing on earth is more debilitating than being cut down in the prime of life by a stroke, the destruction of a portion of the brain caused by a blockage of blood flow to the area. Even a mild attack can leave a man temporarily paralyzed, blind or unable to talk. An estimated 300,000 men suffer strokes each year—and 100,000 will die, according to the National Stroke Association. Doctors say many of these tragedies could be prevented.

Studies show that taking regular doses of aspirin, especially if you have a history of heart or circulation problems, offers significant protection from strokes. Aspirin helps keep arteries from clogging up and blocking blood flow to the brain or heart.

It takes only small doses of aspirin to attain these benefits. "We're talking 30 to 81 milligrams," says New York physician Isadore Rossman, M.D., Ph.D., author of *Looking Forward: The Complete Medical Guide to Successful Aging.* Your pharmacist may stock 81-milligram doses, but if you can't find them, breaking a standard 325-milligram tablet into quarters will give you four correct doses. (Check with your doctor before starting an aspirin regimen.) How often you take aspirin is just as important as how much: Preventive effects are greatest when you take one 81-milligram dose every day or every other day.

In addition to protecting your heart, some studies suggest that taking aspirin regularly can reduce the risk of colon cancer and cataracts, protect against gallstones and boost three important immune-system chemicals.

Since high blood pressure is a major cause of strokes, you can help protect yourself by getting your blood pressure checked as often as possible. A study found that systolic pressure (the top number) is a more accurate predictor of stroke risk than the diastolic reading (the bottom number).

Cut Back on Protein

Your body needs protein for building everything from muscles to bones. Unfortunately, it doesn't need as much as most of us give it.

"The average American eats twice the protein he needs," says Art Mollen, D.O., medical director of the Southwest Health Institute in Phoenix and author of *The Anti-Aging Diet.* An excess of protein can make you feel heavy, sluggish and, over time, physically feeble. Dr. Mollen and others say we'd be better off eating more like the rural Chinese, whose grain-and-vegetable diet is extremely low in animal protein and whose death rate from colon cancer is about 2.5 times lower than ours.

For optimal health, eat 1 gram of protein for every 3 pounds of body weight per day, suggests Dr. Mollen. That's about 50 grams for a 150-pound man. A small portion of sirloin steak trimmed of fat contains about 35 grams, so limit yourself to one protein-based meal per day. "If you have a hamburger for lunch, that's fine, but have cereal or fruit for breakfast and pasta for dinner," says Dr. Mollen.

Drop Pounds, Not Calories

We all want to cut a trim profile around the middle. A lean physique looks better, and more youthful, than a pear-shaped one. Lean men are also more active, more energetic and statistically less prone to chronic debilitating illnesses like diabetes and heart disease. To stay slim, however, men mistakenly tend to cut back on calories when the real villain is lack of exercise and too much fat, says aging researcher Eric Poehlman, Ph.D., of the University of Vermont's Department of Medicine.

In fact, trying to keep weight off simply by cutting calories may not be a smart idea. By eating less, you risk cheating your body of important nutrients, says Dr. Poehlman. His formula for healthy weight loss is to exercise more as you reach middle age and to *eat more calories* as well. Just be sure they're low-fat calories. As a rule of thumb, 60 to 70 percent of your diet should consist of foods high in complex carbohydrates, such as bread, pasta and beans.

Supplement Your Diet

You can protect yourself against both heart disease and cancer by getting more of the powerhouse nutrients vitamins E and C and beta-carotene. All three can reduce your levels of free radicals, damaged molecules that cause harmful changes in the body. One theory holds that the aging process itself is the cumulative result of wear and tear from free radicals.

Unlike many other nutrients, vitamins E and C and beta-carotene are safe to take in amounts higher than the Recommended Dietary Allowance (RDA). "Since the risk is nil, it's safe to take more," says

Jeffrey Blumberg, Ph.D., professor of nutrition at Tufts University. He suggests that optimal intakes for antioxidants may be in the range of 100 to 400 international units of vitamin E, 500 to 1,000 milligrams of vitamin C and 15 to 25 milligrams of beta-carotene every day.

Have Plenty of Sex

Physically, there's no getting around the fact that there's going to be some decrease in the pure animal drive you felt as a teenager. That's partly because, as you leave your teen years, you begin to have more to think about than sex. There is also some slowing down of the basic equipment as the arteries that carry blood to the penis lose flexibility. A regular exercise program can help remedy this by clearing away fatty deposits on arterial walls.

And, while there's no such thing as strength training for the penis, there is an exercise you can do to help keep your erections as firm as possible, says William Hartman, M.D., codirector of the Center for Marital and Sexual Studies in Long Beach, California. The exercise is often called a "Kegel for men," and it works by strengthening the pelvic-floor muscles, the ones situated right beneath the base of the penis. First, find the right muscles: They're the ones you use to stop urine flow. Squeeze the muscles tightly for three seconds, then release. Start from a few and work up to 200 per day.

Just as important as keeping fit is continuing to have sex, not just for physical reasons but for psychological ones as well. "Giving up on sex at any age can be symbolically giving up on all of life," says E. Douglas Whitehead, M.D., a New York urologist specializing in treating impotence. "It can drain vitality out of your marriage, your work, your sense of physical well-being and many of the other satisfactions that the second half of life can bring."

Shun the Sun

Yes, you've heard it. But if you're serious about keeping those youthful good looks of yours, you'd better *do* it. Sun damage is responsible for most of what we think of as aging. Skin damage builds up invisibly for years before you actually see it. In Australia, where men spend lots of time outdoors, scientists find sun damage causes wrinkling as early as age 20.

"The sun damages your skin completely," explains Karen Burke, M.D., of the Scripps Clinic and Research Foundation in La Jolla,

California. "It gradually destroys your skin's inner elastic tissue and breaks down the connective tissue, all causing premature aging. As the outer layer of your skin thickens to protect the vital inner layers, your skin becomes leathery and old looking."

There's also evidence that sunlight may play a role in the formation of gallstones. In a study, the risk of gallstones was 25 times greater for sunburn-prone subjects who sunbathed than for those who didn't. According to one theory, ultraviolet light from the sun, which triggers the skin's pigment system, may lead to an increase of pigments in the bile. This in turn could trigger gallstone formation.

No man is about to stay out of the sun altogether. But while you're out there, protect yourself by wearing a sunscreen with a sun protection factor (SPF) of 15 or higher, advises dermatologist Fredric Haberman, M.D., of Albert Einstein College of Medicine in New York City. "People think they need sunscreen only when they see the sun," Dr. Haberman says. "That's not true. You need it when it's cloudy, too, because clouds don't stop damaging ultraviolet rays." As added protection, he recommends wearing a hat with a brim to block damage from reflected light.

If you've already got wrinkles, you can do some repair work with Retin-A cream. Studies continue to show that regular use of this prescription medicine can eliminate the fine lines around the eyes and soften coarse wrinkles on the upper portions of the face. Dermatologists are now combining Retin-A with alpha hydroxy acids to reduce the irritation and redness that some people experience when they begin to use the medication.

Stand Up to Aging

A hunched-over posture won't cause any medical problems, but it will certainly make you look old before your time. Most posture problems result from bad habits or weak back muscles. Start by fixing the habit: To walk tall, keep your rear tucked in, pull in your chin, tighten your stomach muscles and keep your knees unlocked. Then, if your back muscles are weak or frequently feel stiff, join a health club and ask your health instructor for specific exercises to correct the problem.

For the long term, you also need to guard your bones against loss of calcium. Men lose this mineral more slowly than women do, but we *do* lose it, especially in the spine, says Richard Sprott, Ph.D., who heads the NIA's Biology-of-Aging Program. Too little calcium can eventually make you slouch and can also lead to greater risk of crippling injury. To get enough, experts recommend eating calcium-rich foods such as skim milk, low-fat cheese, low-fat yogurt, broccoli, nuts and dried fruits. Also important is regular exercise, particularly weight training, which makes bones denser and stronger.

Bolster Your Back

One minute you're zooming purposefully out the door on your way to hammer an opponent at racquetball; then you stoop for your gym bag and *boing,* you're instantly a crippled old man who can barely hobble to the nearest chair. "I've had back pain myself, and I can tell you that when you can barely move, and can't play sports or exercise, it profoundly changes your life and your whole sense of well-being," says Alexis P. Shelekov, M.D., a spine surgeon at the Texas Back Institute in Dallas.

Most back troubles are minor problems caused by weak muscles, particularly the abdominals, which provide most of the spine's support. To strengthen them, Dr. Shelekov recommends walking, in conjunction with curl-ups: Lie on your back with your knees bent and your hands on your thighs. Keeping your lower back pressed to the ground, lift your head, neck and shoulders. Hold for a count of two; return. Start with five per day, working up to three sets of ten. As your abdominals become stronger, try the curl-ups with your hands across your chest.

Get Enough Sleep

The legions of sleep-deprived stumble to their desks every morning, dragging themselves through the day fired with coffee and sugar and . . . excuse me, what were we talking about?

"Lack of rest at any age is going to make you *feel* old," says Michael Vitiello, associate director of the Sleep and Aging Research Program at the University of Washington in Seattle. Fatigue makes you physically slow and mentally dull. How much sleep is enough? "It's not so important how long you sleep as how good you feel during the day as a result," says Vitiello. "If you always feel draggy in the morning or late afternoon, you probably need more time in bed." To rest best, he advises turning in and getting up at the same times every day in order to keep your body clock in sync.

Have a Drink

Research continues to pour in showing that moderate drinking (one or two alcoholic drinks per day—no more) protects against heart disease. In fact, drinking men in one recent study had less risk of death from heart disease than men who never touch the stuff.

Alcohol boosts levels of HDL cholesterol (the good kind), "and there are surprisingly few things that'll do that," says Dr. Rossman. Still, doctors are cautious about prescribing alcohol as preventive medicine, since heavy drinking damages the heart, brain and liver. Can you draw the line at a drink or two a day? If not, well, you're a big boy; you're better off saying no.

Stimulate Your Mind

Your brain is not unlike your brawn. Exercise it and it'll get bigger and stronger. There's not much sense working to have the body of a 20-year-old if your mental capacity is slowly sliding toward senility.

Experts say mental challenges can sharpen your thinking. In one four-year study, healthy older people who stayed employed or did volunteer work or gardening had more blood flowing to their brains and did significantly better on IQ tests than less active peers. What's more, research suggests that people whose minds stay sharp into old age also live longer.

To keep your mind stimulated, indulge in hobbies and puzzles that are different from what you do on your job; they'll make your mind work in new ways (and have the added benefit of relaxing you). Socializing of any kind keeps the mind geared up for conversation. Reading a variety of newspapers gives you different perspectives on similar events.

You can also keep your mind fit by keeping your body fit. Long-term aerobic exercise has been shown to help keep older people mentally sharp, according to research at the Medical College of Pennsylvania. A study there found that men age 60 and older who had exercised regularly for five or more years scored significantly higher than nonexercisers of the same age on tests measuring mental quickness and recall.

Live Well

Is aging a state of mind? There's not much science to prove it, but a surprising number of the researchers and doctors we spoke to said that you'll stay young if you think young. Among the benefits mentioned: A positive outlook will help you stick with an exercise program, take an interest in others and stay active longer.

A positive attitude is largely a matter of feeling you have control over your life, says Robin Barr, Ph.D., of the NIA's Adult Psychological Development Program. He points to studies of men in nursing homes who stay healthier and live longer solely by virtue of, for example, being free to find their own way to the lunchroom rather than being taken there.

"In the end, aging is a way of thinking," says Dr. Douglas. "In the past, we've thought that a person was old at age 65. It just isn't the case at all."

—*Richard Laliberte*

Staying Strong

With the right kind of upkeep, your body can be as tough at 50 as it was at 20—maybe tougher. The secret is training smart.

Just because you don't find many over-40 men in those swinging singles health clubs doesn't mean that older guys can't cut the mustard. I see men in their fifties, sixties and even seventies working out all the time, but I usually find them at a bodybuilding gym—the kinds of places with nothing but free weights and musty old leg machines. They're not there to socialize and pose in designer sweats; they're there to work hard and get strong. They know something that's escaped far too many middle-aged Americans: The older you get, the more beneficial strength training is for you.

It's no secret that cardiovascular improvement through aerobic exercise is a life extender and disease preventer. Armed with that knowledge, hordes of older Americans have hit the pavements with walking programs or have put in their time on stationary cycles. They're all the healthier for it.

SETTING THE PACE AT 75

Jerry Wible may be slowing down a bit. Twenty years ago, when he was 55, he could do a standing broad jump of 7 feet, 3 inches. At last year's California Senior Olympics, his best jump was 6 feet, 6 inches. Wible isn't letting this get him down, though. After all, he can still run a mile in under 7 minutes, and he won three medals at the North American Masters Track and Field Championships.

At 5 feet 10 inches and 165 pounds, Wible is in great shape for a man of 75 (or a man of 35). He's up at 5:30 every morning for ten miles of running and walking. If there's a local track meet with a master's category, he'll enter that, or he'll spend some time training for the Senior Olympics. If the ten acres of lawn at his Pennsylvania house need cutting, he does the job with a 21-inch push mower, the kind that runs on human power. When he travels, he always takes his running shoes. "I've run in 100 countries and on every continent," he says.

In addition to exercising daily, Wible watches his diet carefully. "I drink two or three quarts of water a day. No sodas. And I rarely drink alcohol. Not too much red meat and lots of fish. My cholesterol is 152. My resting pulse is 48 to 50."

His doctor is convinced Wible will live to be 100. Wible himself thinks he can do better. "Different articles claim we should be able to live to 125 or 140. Most people just don't take care of themselves."

—*Ricki Stein*

But what about muscles? Once men hit middle age, they tend to shy away from strength training, even though there's no reason in the world *not* to do it and every reason in the world *to* do it. Older men stand to gain all the benefits from a stronger physique that younger men do: better overall health, improved posture, more power and stamina, a more attractive (and, it might be added, a younger-looking) body and, perhaps most important of all, a bolstered self-image that translates into a bright, springy confidence.

"Strength training does add years to your life," says Frederick C. Hatfield, Ph.D., an exercise physiologist who runs the Consortium for Rehabilitation and Fitness Therapy Center in Reseda, California. "It's been proven again and again in recent years. But the main reason that people in their forties and fifties should train isn't for the *length* of their life but for the *quality* of their life. It's one thing to live to be 90 years old, but if you're feeble and helpless, you're not going to enjoy those years. Strength training beats aging by making life more worth living for longer."

Muscles are as able to respond to training in the fifth and sixth decades of life as they are in the third and fourth. Aging doesn't cause significant muscle cell loss. So since the object of weight training is to increase the size of muscle cells, not the number, you have virtually as much to work with at age 50 as you did at 25.

Lifting into the Nineties

A Tufts University study of nursing-home residents who used weight training found that the elderly people were able to increase their strength by as much as 200 percent and their muscle size by up to 15 percent. Even people in their nineties became stronger and increased the size of their muscles after working out on a Universal weight-training machine.

"You see lots of champion-caliber powerlifters who are stronger in their forties and even fifties than ever," says Dr. Hatfield, who counts himself among that group. Dr. Hatfield, now 46, set the world squat record at 1,014 pounds just a few years ago, and he's still competing.

So if building your muscles in your postyouth years helps you beat back the bugaboo of aging, why do so many older men avoid it? The reason probably has to do with the prevailing myth that as you get older, you necessarily get weaker. That's patently untrue, at least up until the age of 60. The fact is that there's less deterioration of muscles than other components of your body as time goes on. The medical community will tell you that until age 60, you'll probably retain 90 percent of your maximum strength—if you use your muscles. "There is some loss of elasticity," says Dr. Hatfield, "so what happens is people get lulled into believing that because they're feeling some changes with age, they can no longer train. That just isn't true. It's disuse, not use, that makes you lose strength in later years."

Actually, Dr. Hatfield contends, those men who have trained throughout their life might find that their workouts can be more and more beneficial as they get older. That's because muscle building is a complex endeavor, and your body responds in myriad ways, some more effective than others. Those in their forties and fifties have learned, perhaps subconsciously, the techniques and approaches that work best for them. They can do it better because they can do it smarter.

"It's like rubbing sandpaper on your hand," says Dr. Hatfield. "Do it one way and you'll get calluses. Do it another and you'll get blisters. Do it regularly for 30 years and you know how to avoid the blisters and get calluses."

The Sooner, the Better

Of course, not everybody pushing 40 has been working out regularly throughout life, and many are concerned that budding middle age is not a safe time to start. Any responsible training advisor would recommend that men over 35 check with their doctor before starting up a weight-training program. It is true that the risk of injury or complications is greater after that age if you train incorrectly. The solution is simple: Train correctly.

"You can't shoot a cannon out of a canoe" is one of Dr. Hatfield's favorite expressions, one he uses with clients such as New York Met Sid Fernandez and sculpted pro football linemen Pete Koch and Mark Gastineau. "You have to build a solid foundation. That's especially true with older trainees, who often want to concentrate on one body part, perhaps thinking they don't have the time for a well-rounded development. That's dangerous.

"For example, even at a very advanced age, you can learn to bench-press 300 pounds. But as you build up just your pectoral muscles to do that, you could blow out your shoulders or arms in the process. Older people especially must start very slowly with a total-body development program, and then work up gradually."

So, does strength training "beat" aging? That is almost as much a philosophical question as a medical one. The modern medical community is nearly unanimous in the belief that regular vigorous exercise combats the kinds of diseases that older Americans are prone to, notably heart disease. Muscleheads like Dr. Hatfield are convinced that weight training adds years—and, of course, better quality—to your life. But nothing stops the clock.

What weight training really does is allow you to make a statement about what your life is going to be like as time passes. Most age-related sacrifices are the result of acquiescing to false notions of what you can or can't do as you get older; the best example of this is allowing your muscles to weaken because of the myth that there's nothing you can do about it.

Everybody has his own physical potential at any age, and the closer you get to it, the better your life will be. If you're 48 and you're hesitant about strength training because "in two years I'll be 50, for heaven's sake," you're cheating yourself. In two years, you're going to be 50 no matter what. It's a question of what kind of 50 you want to be.

—Kelly Garrett

The Muscular Mind

It's not what you've got; it's how you use it. Here's a guide to maximizing your brain power—at any age.

The sun was gleaming through clear Denver skies as United Airlines flight 232 bound for Chicago took off on the afternoon of July 19, 1989. All aboard expected a routine trip. And so it was, until 3:16 P.M., when the tail engine suddenly exploded. Passengers rocked forward and attendants plummeted to the floor as the huge DC-10 pitched downward.

With the two remaining jets under the wings, the plane still had power enough to fly. But power wasn't the problem. The blast had demolished the aircraft's hydraulic system, causing a complete loss of control of the rudder, wing flaps and ailerons. The 296 passengers were trapped at 37,000 feet in a plane with no steering. Captain Alfred C. Haynes had some fast thinking to do.

The situation called for an emergency landing, but the nearest strip was at Iowa's Sioux City Airport, 70 miles away. Although the steering was shot, Captain Haynes found he could maintain some control by alternating speeds of the two wing jets. For 41 minutes, he and his three-man crew struggled to guide the disabled plane closer to the airport. On approach, Captain Haynes shouted through the intercom, "Brace! Brace! Brace!" Moments later the highly unstable aircraft somersaulted to the ground. Miraculously, 184 survived, many without a scratch.

For landing his plane against staggering odds, Captain Haynes was commended for his exceptionally clear thinking and called a national hero, a label he had a hard time accepting. "There is no hero," he said. "There is just a group of four people, four people who did their job."

Perhaps, but by some standards Haynes is overly modest. "If you look at heroes in the movies, it's always the person who knows the right thing to do," says psychologist Dorothy Tennov, Ph.D. "Superman not only had great strength, he also knew how to use it."

While most of the important decisions we make in life are made in less dramatic circumstances than Captain Haynes's, or Superman's for that matter, there are lessons for all of us here. The most important one is that no amount of training can compensate for crystal-clear thinking. Whether your decision concerns an investment, a job, a new house or which set of parents you're going to visit for Easter, clear thinking can help you make the best one.

Clear thinkers aren't born that way. They work at it. Before making important choices, they try to clear emotion, bias, trivia and preconceived notions out of the way so they can concentrate on the information essential to making the right decision.

If your thinking isn't always as focused as you'd like it to be or if you find that you often make choices you later regret, especially if you have to make them quickly, it's time for a course in clear thinking. Here are a few lessons from some of the best-known people in the business.

Assemble the Facts

Before you can make a good decision, you have to assemble all the facts. Not just the obvious stuff, but everything you can get your hands on. Although Captain Haynes's time was extremely limited, he had to gather certain information before he could choose a course of action. How much damage had the explosion caused?

Which controls were still available to him? What sites were open for an emergency landing?

"Mistakes are usually made because someone had insufficient or bad data," says John C. Johnson, M.D., director of emergency medical services at Porter Memorial Hospital in Valparaiso, Indiana.

The way to get good data is to ask questions. At the emergency room, Dr. Johnson is faced with life-or-death crises daily. It's his powers of observation and a willingness to think beyond the obvious that get him through. For example, he describes the case of a badly wheezing child whisked into the emergency room for care. If the attending doctor wasn't thinking clearly, he might reason that the child was having an asthma attack and treat him accordingly. But a sharper doctor would first ascertain when the wheezing began and whether the child had been playing with any small objects. He might discover that the child was choking—and save a life.

As Sherlock Holmes said to the ever-bumbling Watson: "It is a capital mistake to theorize before you have all the evidence. It biases the judgment."

Look under Every Rock for Hidden Opportunities

Take the job/don't take the job. Can't decide? What about other choices? In just about any given situation, a little thinking turns up more options you could take. But if you're like most, you never seek out all these choices. It's easy to get forced into anxiety-ridden "either/or" situations.

One way you may be limiting your options is by springing upon the first solution to a problem that shows itself. But "your first answer is likely not to be your best," says Jeff Salzman, vice-president of CareerTrack, a Colorado-based consulting company. Instead say, "Okay, I have one possible answer—let's see if I can find something better."

The cerebral world of chess offers a perfect example of the importance of creative thinking. According to Michael Valvo, one of America's top-rated chess players, the downfall of many in chess—as in life—is that they "concentrate on only two or three moves while at least seven or eight are usually available."

Keep Your Cool

Imagine what was going through Captain Haynes's mind when he found himself in the cockpit of a crippled plane with the lives of nearly 300 people depending on his judgment. Did he wring his hands? Did he visualize the flaming destruction that could have been moments away?

Of course not. If he had, there'd be no story to tell. "I really didn't have any thoughts," he says. "There was nothing on my mind but what we were trying to accomplish—just the job at hand, which was to bring the plane down safely."

How can you always be coolheaded, especially at a trying moment? The key, our experts agree, is self-confidence.

We know what you're probably thinking: *Easy for us to say*. Sure, Captain Haynes had confidence in his flying skills, but what about decisions that involve whole new sets of parameters you're not familiar with? Having self-confidence can be hard when you lack experience, agrees Dr. Johnson. His advice to young doctors who get hung up trying to decide if they're doing the right thing is to look to the good decisions they have made in the past to reinforce their confidence. There's no reason you can't do the same.

The heart of this issue is trust . . . of yourself. It's an attitude that has at its core an acceptance of yourself and your decisions regardless of what anybody else thinks or any mistakes you may have made, says Albert Ellis, Ph.D., president of the Institute for Rational Emotive Therapy in New York City.

Be an "Amiable Skeptic"

The tough part about being a cool thinker and separating your emotions from your reasoning is that there are lots of people out there who'd rather you remain emotional—like the boss or spouse who uses emotion-inciting ploys to get you to do something you don't want to do. To prevent yourself from being lured into making bad decisions, it's important to view things with a critical eye, says Diane Halpern, Ph.D., a professor of psychology at California State University. That means developing what she calls an attitude of "amiable skepticism." Amiable, because it doesn't entail an adversarial relationship with the world. You can be doubtful and still be cheerful. You can decide to reserve judgment when you sense you're being swayed against your will. It begins with advertising and extends to telephone salesmen offering trips to Hawaii for $300 and all the way to politicians promising to be kinder while they're acting tougher.

Create a Balance Sheet

Whatever decision is looming before you, you want to make the best one. You've already gathered all the information, searched hard to come up with many different avenues. Now it's rating time.

The best way to do it, say the experts, is to grab paper and pen and put together a list of all of the advantages and disadvantages of each option. You can use any rating system you like, but we favor the basic 1-to-10.

Then do some quick arithmetic. "You'll normally find that one option comes out with a distinctly better score," says Dr. Ellis. If you *don't* make such a list, he warns, you risk allowing your emotions to give a disproportionate weight to a single aspect.

He gives as an example a young man he knows who purchased a flashy—but quite undependable—car simply because it turbocharged his ego. Naturally, the guy soon found himself with a car he was kicking more than driving.

Drop Your "Musts"

While in the midst of trying to make a decision, any decision, listen to your inner self. Do you hear a cranky little voice inside saying, "I must have this . . . I must . . . I must . . . I *must!*" People are born with a tendency to take their important desires and turn them into "musts," says Dr. Ellis.

The problem is that this limits your ability to think in an objective manner. The key to rational thinking and clear decision making is to remain flexible. So the next time you hear yourself saying "I *must!*" step back and ask yourself, *"Must* I?" Ask yourself if the sabbatical you've been fantasizing about taking really makes more sense after the kids get out of college; consider whether a dependable car might make more sense than that Porsche 911 you saw at the used-car lot. You might be surprised how good it feels to make the more logical (read: grown-up) choice.

Chop Up Big Decisions

A big decision can be like an enormous chunk of steak. Try to swallow it without first cutting it up, and you risk choking. So says

Paul Slovic, Ph.D., professor of psychology at the University of Oregon and president of Decision Research, a nonprofit research institute in Eugene, who recommends a technique he calls "incrementalism." Say, for instance, that you're considering giving up your job as a salesman in Chicago to become a sportswriter in Miami. The decision involves not only starting a new career but also selling your house, moving your family and leaving all your friends. You've been agonizing over this one for some time.

Decisions like this can be overwhelming, says Dr. Slovic. The thing to do if you feel overwhelmed is to cut up the dilemma into smaller pieces. Perhaps you can find a part-time newspaper job in Chicago, while keeping your present job, to see if reporting will be as much to your liking as you think. Possibly you can take time off from work and spend it in Miami with the family, to see how much everyone goes for Florida living. You may be surprised. "We tend to think that we can predict new situations better than we actually can," says Dr. Slovic.

Get a Second Opinion

When time allows, it's a good idea to consult with other people before making important decisions. There are just too many things in this world that are too big for any one person to examine alone.

But whose opinion do you ask? You could go to your best friend or someone else with whom you share common interests and values. But you'll do much better by asking people who think differently. People who are like you will probably agree with you. That'll boost your confidence, but not the accuracy of the decision.

A better tactic is to go to people with different backgrounds, different occupations—different biases. And if you want to get double your money's worth from a second opinion, ask for it before you reveal your own feelings, say the experts. Don't walk in and say, "I've decided that I'm going to get this operation—what do *you* think?" The advice you get will be much more valuable if it comes without any influence from you.

Don't Rush the Verdict

The old advice "Sleep on it" makes a lot of sense. Your opinions will be more valuable if you harvest them after allowing them time to ripen. Your vision becomes clearer over time about decisions and judgments you need to make.

There's a good reason for this. "We're heavily influenced by recency," says Donald A. Norman, Ph.D., a professor of cognitive science at the University of California in San Diego. For instance, if you had to travel to London two days after a major airline crash, you might seriously think about canceling the trip. "Leaving a little time to put recent things in the past can help a lot to clarify thinking," he says.

Prove Yourself Wrong

Most of us, when we make up our mind, set out immediately to validate what we think we "know," states Dr. Ellis. As time goes on, we find more and more "proof" that our assumptions are correct because all we're looking for is that proof. "But we tend to learn more by trying to falsify our assumptions," says Dr. Ellis.

There's no better way to find holes in the fabric of faulty thinking than to ask yourself, "What are the reasons I may be wrong?" Try asking this question of yourself the next time you feel absolutely sure about something. You've got nothing to lose but your possible error!

—*Russell Wild*

Take Two Risks and Call Me in the Morning

There's nothing more empowering for a man than to meet his fears and overcome them. So take some risks now and then. The doctor says it will be good for you.

By most accounts, my college roommate was a conservative fellow. He voted for Reagan, preferred playing the piano to partying
(continued on page 23)

HOW GUTSY ARE YOU?

Are you an adventure-loving kind of guy, or is your idea of a big risk not guaranteeing a hotel room for late arrival? Is there a thrill seeker hidden inside that buttoned-down exterior of yours? Take this quiz to measure your risk quotient and see if you're a Milquetoast or a maniac.

There are no right or wrong answers here. Nor is any score better than another. Circle only one letter per question. Answer all questions. If no answer feels exactly right to you, pick the one that's closest. To determine your score, total all numbers circled and see "Scoring," on page 23.

1. During the past ten years, how often have you changed residence?
   a. 10 times or more
   b. 5–9 times
   c. 2–4 times
   d. 0–1 times

2. Which adjective best describes your behavior before age 12?
   a. hyperactive
   b. mischievous
   c. basically well behaved
   d. very well behaved

3. In an average week, how many hours of TV do you watch?
   a. 0–5
   b. 6–10
   c. 11–20
   d. more than 20

4. How often do you tape shut already-sealed envelopes before mailing them?
   a. almost never
   b. seldom
   c. often
   d. regularly

5. When eating Chinese food, how often do you use chopsticks?
   a. almost never
   b. seldom
   c. often
   d. regularly

6. In highway driving, how often do you drive faster than 65 mph?
   a. regularly
   b. often
   c. seldom
   d. almost never

7. If you were living on the East Coast a century ago, do you think you would have joined a wagon train headed west?
   a. definitely
   b. probably
   c. probably not
   d. definitely not

8. Suppose you had equal competence at any one of the following activities. Which would appeal to you most?
   a. skydiving
   b. mountain climbing
   c. producing a play
   d. building a house

Assume that you are equally capable at all of the activities listed below. For each set, pick the one that you would most enjoy. (If neither activity appeals to you, pick the one that's less unappealing.)

9. a. driving a dune buggy
   b. hiking in the desert

10. a. skiing down a steep slope
    b. ski touring through woods

11. a. scuba diving
    b. snorkeling

Circle the letter of the word that best describes your reaction to the following activities.

12. Building a cabinet
    a. tedious
    b. satisfying

(continued)

HOW GUTSY ARE YOU?—CONTINUED

13. Climbing rocks
    a. exhilarating
    b. scary

14. Attending a rock concert
    a. arousing
    b. jarring

15. Teaching school
    a. boring
    b. challenging

16. With a report due at work in two weeks, would you be most likely to:
    a. start working on it the day before it's due, then stay up most of the night completing it
    b. work hard on the report for a day or two before it's due
    c. start working on it during the second week
    d. budget time throughout the two weeks to produce the report

17. In general, do you prefer the company of:
    a. people you've recently met
    b. professional colleagues, coworkers or fellow members of a club or church

18. Which opportunity sounds more appealing to you?
    a. starting your own business
    b. purchasing a successful business

19. Which statement describes you better?
    a. I get bored easily.
    b. When necessary, I can tolerate routine.

20. What kinds of risks would you say are hardest for you to take?
    a. commitment risks (ones involving long-term involvement with a person, faith, activity or career)
    b. emotional risks (in relationships, or showing my feelings)
    c. financial risks (of losing money)
    d. physical risks (of life and limb)

Scoring: Give yourself 1 point for each *a*, 2 points for each *b*, 3 for each *c* and 4 for each *d*.

30 or below: Suggests a high need for excitement and a low tolerance for boredom. You're more likely than other men to take physical risks and to avoid emotional or long-term commitments. You're best suited to jobs that involve constant crises, such as emergency-room doctor, commodities trader or small-business owner. Potential problems: reckless driving, drug and alcohol abuse, compulsive gambling.

31 and above: Suggests you find it hard to take physical and financial risks, but easy to take long-term risks such as deciding to raise a family or committing yourself to a career. Tolerance for routine and ability to take the long view make you ideal for management or supervisory jobs. Potential problems: lethargy and depression.

and was usually asleep by 11:00 P.M. He appeared to be the embodiment of dullness and predictability. But one Saturday morning, while I was still in bed trying to determine the molecular weight of a can of Budweiser, he burst into the room with a smug grin on his face. "I just jumped out of a plane at 10,000 feet," he said. "I'm going to do it again tomorrow. Wanna try it?"

I politely declined. I've never been that crazy about the idea of riding in airplanes, let alone leaping out of them. What if the guy who packed my parachute had a really bad hangover that day? What if I drifted into a high-tension power line and got roasted? What if I landed in the lagoon of a sewage treatment plant and drowned? Hadn't I read about that happening to someone a few years ago?

I think I know why my buddy did something so seemingly uncharacteristic, perhaps even foolhardy. He did it *because* it was uncharacteristic and foolhardy. He needed to travel to the edge and dance on it for a while because his life was so otherwise boring and predictable.

Everyone needs some of that risk and excitement. After all, in terms of evolution, we've been wearing suits and living in split-levels for only a speck of time. Most of our prehistoric past was filled with uncertainty, danger and extreme risks. The people who survived were those who thrived on those risks. We're their heirs, and that need for a certain amount of risk is still strong in us.

I don't need airplanes and parachutes to fulfill my adventure quotient; roller coasters do it for me. I get sweaty palms and a flip-flopping stomach just waiting in line. Being strapped in the seat is exquisite agony. By the time I reach the top of the first steep rise, I'm convinced that death is moments away. My heart is in my mouth through the entire ride. When it's over, I feel . . . terrific. I've spit in the eye of fear, grabbed myself an energizing jolt of adrenaline.

Risk Builds Character

Not only is this fun, it's good for me. Experts who have studied risk taking say it develops character and courage, extends creativity, boosts confidence and helps establish a sense of limitations and possibilities. They say that if you don't allow yourself some conscious risks, you may be more likely to take unconscious ones such as driving too fast, drinking too much, picking fights or gambling away money, relationships or a job.

"It's important to take risks to experience life," says Frank Farley, Ph.D., a psychologist at the University of Wisconsin. "If you don't expose yourself to new experiences and new ideas, you remain the same. And change is a very important part of personal growth."

Farley, who coined the term *T-Type personality* to describe people who love risks, says you don't have to run out and sign up for a course in rattlesnake wrestling to get a charge. "Anytime you can overcome a fear or meet a challenge and not run from it, it strengthens you as a person," he says. Dr. Farley considers healthy risk taking to be anything to which the outcome is uncertain. This includes not only obvious stuff like bungee jumping and rock climbing but also psychological and financial risks like starting a business, investing in the stock market or changing careers.

In fact, only the risk taker himself can determine what's risky. Some of us choose to take risks in one part of our lives but not in another. The defining element is fear. There's no thrill—and no real risk—without that. When Phillipe Petit, the acrobat who walked a wire between the World Trade Center towers, was asked about his feat, he said that balancing 110 stories above ground without a net wasn't all that scary for him.

What did he consider risky?

Spiders, snakes . . . and getting married, he replied. He'd rather do 10,000 backward somersaults on a high wire than get married and have kids.

Fear of Failing

Fear is what makes us avoid risk, makes us run away from challenges, play it safe. We do it to spare ourselves failure, embarrassment, bankruptcy, injury or death. But, says Dr. Farley, "There's nothing more empowering for a man than to meet his fears and overcome them." His studies show that risk takers are more self-confident, energetic, creative and independent than less daring men.

In nearly every high-risk sport, the mastery of fear comes up repeatedly as the principal reward for engaging in it. The deeper the fear, the bigger the thrill when you conquer it. One study found that the more frightened sky divers were while going up in a plane, the more exhilarated they felt when they parachuted safely to the ground.

According to Ralph Keyes, author of the book *Chancing It: Why We Take Risks,* that rush is delivered by natural opiate-like body chemicals that kick in during a stressful experience. "It's nature's way of rewarding us for taking chances," he says.

Keyes, who interviewed nearly a thousand T-Types for his book, says some people become addicted to that chemical kick and look for ever-more-challenging ways to keep it coming. A predisposition to thrill seeking, he adds, may even be genetic.

The Foreign Legion?

So maybe you're the kind of guy who likes to avoid the unexpected. You always keep a spare car key in a magnetic case under your bumper. You never leave the house without an umbrella. You wouldn't dream of tearing the label off a mattress. You know you're stuck in an unexciting rut, but you don't know what to do about it. Should you take up hang gliding? Plan a scuba trip to the shark feeding grounds off the Great Barrier Reef?

Probably not, says Dr. Farley. "Many men dream of breaking out of their everyday roles and becoming super-risk-taking heroes overnight, but it doesn't happen very often," he says. "You change by taking small steps into the unknown."

He suggests starting with minor changes. Identify some of your long-held fears and begin pushing them. If you're a creature of habit who always eats at the same restaurants, make it a point to try some new ones. Instead of going on your usual vacation, ask your travel agent about adventure packages. Add variety to your sex life by experimenting with new places and positions. If you can't face a fear head on, try taking risks in another part of your life. "I've always wanted to be a stand-up comic, but I could never get up the nerve," admits Keyes. "Instead I went rock climbing and risked my neck. It was scary, but I was less frightened of that than of getting booed off a stage."

Given the lack of objective standards, how do you decide if a risk is worth taking? Ask yourself what you have to gain if you're successful and what you have to lose if you're not. Dabbling in the stock market is an acceptable risk if you have a few spare dollars; learning to drive a race car with a certified instructor is more likely to thrill you than kill you. On the other hand, going for a spin in your Delta 88 when you've got a bellyful of wine is just dangerous and stupid. (Dr. Farley calls drinking and driving and other purely reckless behaviors T-negative.)

What if you take a risk and fail? Big deal. According to Keyes, the biggest losers are those who never took risks in the first place. He tells of a sky diver who spent a year in the hospital after falling 2,000 feet when his chute failed to open. "Sure, he regretted the accident, but he didn't regret skydiving, and he was ready to go up again." Likewise, people who start businesses that fail, audition for parts they don't get or become deeply involved in relationships that don't pan out are usually proud of themselves for making the effort. "There's a sense of satisfaction in taking a risk—win or lose—that can't be found any other way," Keyes says. "People who choose *not* to take important risks often have deep regrets, almost to the point of mourning."

—*Dan Bensimhon*

The Appearance of Youth

Some hair and skin care advances offer hope, others, just hype. Can you tell them apart?

Probably no signs of aging bother a man more than the ones that show above the shirt collar. Wrinkles, bags under the eyes, a hairline that's heading north—all visible signs to himself and others that the years are sneaking by. And forget what you've heard about The New Male Vanity; this stuff has been bugging men for centuries. In 4000 B.C., Egyptian men were rubbing ground animal parts on their heads in an attempt to grow hair. That dumb wreath that Caesar wore was an early attempt at a toupee. John D. Rockefeller reportedly had a supply of fresh mother's milk delivered daily in the belief that it would keep his skin immune to aging.

The fact that, in the past, none of the miracle cures has ever proven to be more than snake oil has left many men resigned to a life of wearing hats and avoiding mirrors. Ironically, science is just now beginning to deliver on some of those broken promises. Researchers have been chipping away at the problems of wrinkling skin and disappearing hair for decades, and finally there are some strategies and even medicines that offer an alternative to growing old ungracefully.

The Hair Facts

First, let's look at what's happening on the front lines of hair restoration. Most men who lose their hair do so because they are genetically programmed to. Male pattern baldness is a trait that can be inherited from both parents. How it's passed on seems almost random. In many families, one son goes bald and the other does not.

If a man has a genetic predisposition to baldness, the rate of hair loss depends on his age and male sex hormones. Ten percent of men show obvious hair loss in their teens, 20 percent in their twenties, 30 percent in their thirties and so on. Men who become substantially bald usually show significant hair loss by age 35.

Right now, the best treatment for male pattern baldness is the drug minoxidil, sold in the United States under the brand name Rogaine. After a long period of Food and Drug Administration (FDA) scrunity, minoxidil was approved as the first medical treatment for baldness. It appears to work by opening blood vessels in the scalp, which had been too constricted for hair to grow.

In all the hype and hoopla over the discovery and approval of the drug, however, some men may have gotten the impression that it can work miracles. In most cases, it can't.

"The truth about this drug is that it will turn out to be great for some men but a huge disappointment for others," says Harry L. Roth, M.D., a clinical professor of dermatology at the University of California at San Francisco. Dr. Roth directed one of the 27 different year-long studies (involving 2,300 men) that were responsible for earning minoxidil its government approval. "It's important that men be forewarned of what minoxidil can and can't do, and for whom," Dr. Roth says. "Men who are older than 35 and whose baldness is quite extensive will not do well. The drug is most effective for men in their early twenties and thirties whose hair loss has started only within the past several years and is not advanced."

Elise Olsen, M.D., an assistant professor of medicine at the Duke University Medical Center who also directed an FDA minoxidil trial, agrees with Dr. Roth. "Men who have bald areas on the tops of their heads measuring two inches in diameter or less are the ones who will do best with this drug," Dr. Olsen says. "I would be reluctant to prescribe it for men whose conditions are considerably more advanced than that, unless of course their goal would be just to slow down their hair loss."

And indeed, even though minoxidil may not turn out to be the great baldness buster hoped for when this blood pressure drug's hair-raising powers were accidentally discovered more than 15 years ago, the stuff stands a good chance of at least being called a hair saver, which is certainly no small claim in its own right. "This could very well turn out to be minoxidil's greatest contribution," Dr. Roth says. "The FDA's studies did not examine this feature of minoxidil specifically, but the effect was widely observed. Even in men who saw no actual growth from minoxidil, most said they felt it at least slowed down their hair loss."

Other experts agree with the better-for-slowing-than-growing assessment. "The drug is clearly better for retarding hair loss than for growing new hair," says Gene T. Izuno, M.D., dermatologist at the Scripps Clinic in La Jolla, California, where another of the FDA's minoxidil trials was conducted. And according to Dominic Brandy, M.D., medical director of the Cosmetic Hair Replacement Surgery Center in Pittsburgh, "I will be prescribing minoxidil more as a defense against baldness than as a cure for it."

But of course, even already bald men will be coming to minoxidil with hope. Here are the facts they should be aware of when they do.

• Minoxidil works best on men younger than 30 whose hair loss is not extensive and has started only recently, preferably within the past five years. Even among these prime candidates, only one-third can expect good results (at least a doubling in hair density), while about 40 percent can expect fair results (hair thickness doubling and a bald spot that will shrink but not disappear). The others will experience virtually no change, though they may experience a retarding of hair loss.

• Minoxidil cannot grow new hair where there is none. It can only thicken and lengthen existing hairs.

• Minoxidil won't do anything for a receding hairline; it cannot grow hair at the temples or forehead. It works best on bald spots on the top of the head measuring two inches in diameter or less.

• Minoxidil must be applied twice daily for at least four to six months, and sometimes for a full year, before results are seen. A year's supply costs about $700.

• Minoxidil requires a lifetime commitment. A man who stops using it will lose whatever hair he has gained within about six months.

One thing is for sure: Minoxidil will not be the last word in medical treatments for baldness. The potential earnings from a real cure are mind-boggling, and every pharmaceutical company would love a piece. Research continues at a strong pace. (See "Beyond Minoxidil" on page 30.)

If you simply can't wait for science to get around to a dramatic cure, there are alternatives. "If a man is truly committed to having a significantly fuller head of hair, he can have it," says Dr. Brandy. Here's a quick rundown of procedures available.

The hair lift. Most recent and dramatic of the surgical alternatives is the hair lift. In a series of three or four operations, bald scalp is removed, and scalp with hair is moved from the back and sides of the head to the top of the head. Results can be truly remarkable. Depending on how many operations are needed, costs range from $3,000 to $15,000.

BEYOND MINOXIDIL

Minoxidil is the first medical treatment for baldness, but it won't be the last. A number of medications are currently under investigation. All of the drugs are biologic response modifiers, which means that, like minoxidil, they affect the basic control mechanisms of hair follicle development. None of the new agents can cause growth of new hair from follicles that have become defunct, however. All, like minoxidil, require a living hair follicle capable of stimulation. Here's a quick rundown of the drugs presently receiving the most attention. None has yet received FDA approval.

Viprostol. An antihypertensive agent whose effects thus far appear to be similar to, though slightly less dramatic than, minoxidil's.

Diazoxide. A potent antihypertensive and blood vessel dilator that some research has shown to be twice as effective as minoxidil.

Minoxidil plus Retin-A. A mixture that some studies suggest works better than minoxidil alone. The most important factor regarding minoxidil's efficacy seems to be how well it penetrates the scalp, and retinoic acid may improve that penetration, says Edward Bondi, M.D., of the University of Pennsylvania. Retin-A may also have some hair-stimulating properties by itself, according to some researchers.

Scalp reduction. Scalp reduction removes a section of bald scalp from the top of the head as sides are drawn upward to minimize the size of the bald area. It's used when the bald spot is not large enough to warrant a full hair lift. Several operations can be performed a few months apart, the result being a reduction in the bald area. Prices for the procedure range from $500 to $2,000 per operation.

Hair transplants. The procedure, which has been around for over 30 years, takes plugs of hair from the back and sides of the head and surgically embeds them where hair is lacking. Plugs can vary in size from fairly large (8 to 20 hairs) to very small, some consisting of a single hair. Bad hair transplants are a very common problem, according to Dr.

Brandy. "I've seen hundreds of bad transplants in consultation, and I do a lot of repair work. A thorough job requires three or four operations. Otherwise, what you end up with looks like corn rows or picket fences." Prices range from $10 to $40 a plug, with a complete job costing about $6,000, depending on how many plugs are required.

Hair weaving. The procedure is not surgical but merely cosmetic in that it attaches extensions, either natural or synthetic, to existing hairs. On the downside, the extensions must be repositioned every four to six weeks as the hair grows out.

Hairpieces. Toupees seem to be out of favor with baby boomers. Hairpieces have gotten a bad name because so many men wear cheap ones that make them look as if a weasel died on top of their head. It's very hard to spot a good toupee, but the dreadful ones get noticed.

If you're thinking about a hairpiece, your best bet is to go to someone who makes a free consultation. Your best option is a custom piece rather than an off-the-rack toupee. Synthetic pieces are better for active, sports-minded men because they hold up to weather and water better and are easier to keep clean. Natural pieces do tend to look slightly better at first, but the harsh processing done to Oriental hair—the largest hair source—makes the hair break down sooner. As for comparative costs, figure about $150 more for a natural piece than a synthetic piece in the $1,000 category.

Surface Appearance

When it comes to their skin, men have an advantage over women. A man's skin is thicker, so it's less likely to wrinkle. But we're hardly immune. For the better part of three decades, our skin seems ageless. Then, slowly but surely—more slowly in some men than in others—tiny changes occur. The skin begins to lose its immunity to outside irritants. Sweat glands shrink, oil glands become less active and we lose the benefit of their moisturizing capabilities. Wrinkles begin to form. They start where the skin is thinnest—around the eyes. Later, deeper wrinkles appear on the forehead and cheeks.

The degree to which you wrinkle is partly a matter of genetics. But only a small part of it is inevitable. In many cases, the skin breaks down because of photoaging—damage caused by too much exposure to the sun. The effect of this damage over a period of years is what many people think of as aged skin—blotchy, lined and leathery, with reduced elasticity. One of the most dramatic examples of sun damage

I've ever seen was illustrated on a segment of the television show "20/20" last year. Cohost Hugh Downs showed pictures of an Indian woman who had spent most of her life outdoors side by side with those of a Tibetan monk who'd lived indoors for decades. She looked about 92 and he looked about 64. But he was 92 and she was 64.

"You don't have to be sunning for your skin to suffer the photoaging effects of the sun's ultraviolet rays," says Lorraine Kligman, Ph.D., assistant research professor in the Department of Dermatology at the University of Pennsylvania School of Medicine. "Photoaging occurs even when you're walking around doing your normal activities."

The answer isn't to become a monk, though. "Evidence suggests that if you start protecting your skin daily with a broad-spectrum sunscreen, skin that is already damaged will begin to repair itself," says Dr. Kligman. "Much of this repair work won't be visible for a long time. What you will see, however, is that your skin's blotchiness may tend to fade."

Dr. Kligman recommends that you wear a sunscreen with a sun protection factor (SPF) of 15 at all times. An SPF of 15 means that 15 hours in the sun will only add up to the damage that would occur in 1 hour if you were unprotected.

When you're on a fishing trip or doing anything else that keeps you out in intense sunlight for several hours, keep your nose and cheeks covered with zinc oxide cream, which will block nearly all the sun's rays.

Next to the sun, nothing will make you look old before your time quicker than smoking cigarettes will. Any experienced dermatologist will tell you he can spot a smoker at ten yards by his "smoker's face"—heavy wrinkles around the eyes and mouth, poor skin tone and gray pallor. Many doctors say they can see skin damage from smoking in men younger than 30.

Nicotine decreases blood flow to the skin by constricting vessels, and it inhibits the flow of nutrients to the cells of the skin. Tobacco also uses up vitamin C, a nutrient that's crucial to a healthy skin.

Beyond good care, there's always plastic surgery. More men are going under the knife than ever before, although surgery should probably be a last resort. A good face lift can cost $10,000 and require you to miss several weeks of work.

—Paul Neimark

Aging Gracefully, Inside and Out

He's old enough to be playing Grandpa, but Hollywood (and most of America) still thinks he's sexy. Here's the verdict on Paul Newman.

You can't talk about how men stay young without talking about Paul Newman, even if Paul Newman doesn't want to talk about it.

I mean, does this guy look like he was born in 1925? He's 13 years older than Redford, but he's got fewer wrinkles. He's 3 years older than George C. Scott, but Newman doesn't look nearly timeworn enough to pull off those presidential parts that Scott gets. In fact, he still gets to play romantic leads with women who are decades younger.

It's not just those lit-from-within blue eyes, either, although they certainly don't hurt his looks. If Newman were bald and jowly, the eyes might pull him through. But the point is, he's *not* bald or jowly, so the eyes are just a bonus.

My assignment was to find out how Newman does it. How has he managed to look and act so youthful at an age when many men begin to feel old? I figured Newman must have a lot of insight into this. Clearly he thinks about it, since men don't age this gracefully without some effort. I figured he and I would sit down for a chat and I'd pick his brain for a little advice the rest of us can use. We live in the same town (Westport, Connecticut), so it wouldn't be a problem to drive on over to his place—a Revolutionary War–era farmhouse on 11 acres—for a Budweiser and some chat. Maybe he'd even offer a bowl of his famous popcorn to help me work up a thirst.

A call to Newman's public relations people put a quick end to that notion. The word came back from Newman that he didn't want to talk. He said he's "tired of being portrayed as the perennially youthful man."

We should all have such problems. I can't actually recall anyone ever calling me a perennially youthful man, but if someone did, I guarantee I wouldn't get tired of it for a long time.

But okay, I can understand his feelings. Newman's reached an age where he wants to be appreciated for his work as a serious actor, not as a hunk of meat. He eschews vanity and the whole Hollywood thing. And after all, this is a guy who can't go out in public without some lady stopping him and saying, "Take off your sunglasses, I want to see your blue eyes." (These encounters, he has said, continue to annoy him, even after all these years: "It's like saying to a woman, 'Open your blouse, I want to see your chest.' ") But public postures aside, the man *is* perennially youthful, even if he's tired of being reminded, and I suspected he works damned hard at it.

My approach to getting the story was going to have to change, though. Instead of getting it directly from the source, I was going to have to read everything about the man I could get my hands on, talk to his friends and business associates and make a few educated guesses.

No Need for Touched-Up Photos

First, I wanted to establish that Newman's youthful looks weren't achieved by makeup, photo retouching or some other movie magic. Nope, his friends say, he looks that good at the grocery store on Saturday morning, too. Every single one told me he doesn't look *nearly* his age. I heard descriptions like "reed-thin," "almost perfectly proportioned," "holds himself ramrod straight." His height may be debatable (5 feet 10 inches is the official word, although some wags in the tabloid world claim he's shorter), but the wise-guy half-smile and see-through-you blue eyes are incontrovertible. Sure, his family calls him Old Skinny Legs, the hair has gone silver, and little lines are starting to appear below his mouth, but according to Howard Pearson, M.D., medical director of Newman's Hole in the Wall Gang Camp and professor of pediatrics at Yale University School of Medicine, the actor is "lean, hasn't lost his hair, and has an excellent complexion."

Don Kulowski, president of Century Pools in New Britain, Connecticut, and the guy who installed the big pool at Newman's camp, views the actor with admiration and envy. "He's in excellent shape. He's slight, not overweight, and appears to have nonstop energy. He looks like he's in his forties. I'm ten years behind him, and I'd like to be in that kind of shape."

As for the reasons, heredity certainly plays a starring role. Newman is the recipient of a good set of genes. If you saw those magazine ads his older brother, Arthur, did for an investment company, you know that youthful looks run in the family.

Getting good genes is lucky. Excellent physical shape is work. Newman works. Buddy Dinan, the owner of Westport Pool and Spa, has installed two hot tubs and a spa for the Newmans. He says the Blue-Eyed One "swims laps, jogs a lot and does a daily Danish plunge: from sauna to hot tub to cold tub." Dinan sees in Newman, besides a "friendly guy, great to deal with, not aloof," a man with a "strong commitment to life and staying healthy."

Besides the swimming, jogging and saunas, Newman works out on an exercise bike and weight machines every day while watching cable news. Because he has a tendency toward a beer gut, he also does a lot of sit-ups on a slant board. A few years ago, he did so many he gave himself a hernia.

Peter Bush, a Connecticut disc jockey who's been involved in sports car–racing promotions with Newman, describes the actor as being in "exceptional condition for someone his age. He's a classic case of 'You think young, you are young.' He works out regularly, and he makes sure all his parts check out. He has the reaction time of someone much younger."

"He's physically fit," agrees Peter Slater, vice-president of the Newman-Sharp Racing Team, adding that for what an endurance racer goes through, Newman had better be. According to Slater, it's fairly unusual for a man in his sixties to be this good, but Newman still has what it takes: dexterity, coordination, concentration, the ability to handle stress.

About the only aspect of Newman's health regimen with an aura of mystery about it is the ice. *Life* magazine says he "believes in the mysterious preservative powers of ice—in healing and in tightening skin"—and that he likes to dunk his face in a sink of ice cubes for a few seconds every morning. Nuh-uh, says the *New York Times Magazine:* Just a rumor.

Avoiding Dietary Sins

In keeping with the anti-star, regular-guy image that's so important to him, Newman—at least in public—is not a fussy eater. At the racetrack, he'll grab a convenience-store lunch of a ready-made sandwich and grape soda pop. While directing, he'll nosh on salty popcorn from a plastic garbage bag. And he's been known to stop by the Westport Häagen-Dazs occasionally for a vanilla ice-cream bar with milk chocolate and peanuts, although perhaps less often since the time a fellow customer got so flustered at coming face-to-face with

Newman's baby blues that she put her ice cream cone into her pocket-book before exiting.

Although none of the above qualifies as a dietary sin, Newman's real care and feeding habits are more in evidence in his private life. And *here* we see a man who cares about *food*. For years he gave a vinaigrette salad dressing of his own concoction to his best friends as Christmas gifts. Eventually he created Newman's Own, an all-natural line of foods with Newman's Own Salad Dressing as the headliner (supported by spaghetti sauce, popcorn and lemonade). Newman is a man who as often as not dons the chef's toque in his own family (his daughter Nell calls him a "risk taker—with almost flawless results") and won't think twice about driving out for fresh ingredients for his specialties. A man who, with best buddy A. E. Hotchner, well-known writer and fellow Westporter, coauthored *Newman's Own Cookbook*.

Newman "eats lightly," according to Dr. Howard Pearson, who remembers a recent Newman meal of tiny clams on the half shell, angel hair pasta, and scrod with capers. The clam dish is a favorite Newman appetizer; he describes it with loving precision in his cook-book: "A dozen tiny clams on the half shell, topped with a squirt of lemon juice and a dollop of fresh horseradish—but *never* that dread spicy-catsup cocktail sauce! If baby clams are not available, I'll settle for a plate of celery hearts chopped fine in an oil-and-vinegar dressing, which I concoct." His favorite sandwich reportedly is sliced cucumbers on whole wheat.

Newman's only habit that could conceivably be considered a potential vice is the ubiquitous Bud. "If Budweiser went out of business," says Don Kulowski, "Newman would go out of business." On the other hand, Newman hasn't touched hard liquor for years, and there's some evidence that moderate drinking may actually be a healthy habit: A study from the Institute for Aerobics Research in Dallas, for example, has shown that moderate quantities of alcohol seem to lower the risk of heart disease; other studies show a tipple now and then can contribute to longer life. An occasional wine or beer also can mildly sedate the day's jitters and bolster emotional well-being—both important in staving off aging.

Feeling Good by Doing Good

When you think about secrets of graceful aging, you think in terms of fitness, diet, genes—and "other." It's obvious that Newman does pretty well on the first three. Where he really hits the jackpot is in the "other." Newman's at a stage and status in life where he could easily sit back; instead, he's *giving* back. As in doing unto others. As in altruism. And doctors and researchers are now finding that people with an altruistic spirit tend to stay healthier and live longer. The converse of this seems to be true, too: According to research done by Larry Scherwitz, Ph.D., at the Medical Research Institute of San Francisco, self-centered people are much more likely to die of a heart attack than less self-centered people.

Altruism is the main ingredient in Newman's Own. Almost everyone knows that venture started as a goof; not everyone knows it's now a multimillion-dollar business that plows *all* its profits into charity. The American Foundation for AIDS Research, the Cystic Fibrosis Foundation, the American Ballet Theatre, the Central Park Conservancy and the Scott Newman Foundation (named for his son, who reportedly died of an accidental overdose of alcohol and drugs) all have benefited from Newman's generosity.

The main beneficiary these days is Newman's Hole in the Wall Gang Camp, which opened last summer in Ashford, Connecticut. It's a summer camp for kids from 7 to 17 who have cancer or potentially fatal blood diseases. "The idea for the camp was just there, full-blown, one morning," Newman says. "I've had friends who died young. Life is whimsical. Longevity is an incredible gift, and some people don't get to enjoy it."

According to Dr. Pearson, Newman's presence was nothing like "the general view we have of the celebrity who gives to philanthropic causes, the one who comes to the tux-and-black-tie kickoff and then runs out." Dr. Pearson says Newman "oversaw every aspect, from the site selection to the architectural design to the landscaping and the furnishings in the cabins. He took an intimate and continuing part. If there was a meeting with the septic-tank people, he'd be there!"

Kulowski marvels at the way Newman mobilized and motivated all the disparate contractors who pitched in at the Hole in the Wall Gang Camp: "He'd give each his undivided attention—for 90 seconds." Kulowski says Newman made a point of having a few beers with the guys on the construction crew and found a way to make everyone feel important. Peter Bush says it's involvement in causes like the camp that allows Newman to be at peace with himself: "His endless dedication to charitable causes makes him want to wake up every morning and look at the bright side."

Family Ties

The image I like best is Newman as family man. His relationship with Joanne Woodward is by all accounts a solid one after more than 30 years of marriage. Newman has five daughters: Susan and Stephanie from his first marriage to actress Jackie Witte, and Nell, Melissa and Clea with Woodward. Although he gives himself only one thumb-up as Dad, it's clear from the people around him that nothing means more to him than his family. Sometime costar and young sidekick Tom Cruise wraps it nicely: "He lives a normal life. He's got several businesses, a wife, a family. That's good for me to see."

Loving family, devoted friends—another big longevity-plus for Newman. Scientists are pretty confident that the more socially isolated a man is, the less healthy he is psychologically and physically, and the more likely he is to die. Conversely, they suggest, the better his social and family relationships, the longer he's likely to live.

Then there's Newman's sense of humor. Doctors say the ability to have a good laugh is very good for you. It's obvious from the Newman's Own product literature, and from just about every interview the actor has ever given, that he doesn't take himself very seriously. He's said to love a good prank and to be a willing audience for even the corniest joke. As Lindsay Crouse, an actress who worked with Newman on a couple of films, once told an interviewer: "After a serious scene, I'll say to him, 'Hey Paul, you hear the one about . . . ?' Then I tell him the last joke I heard, and no matter how bad it is, he's the best audience. The *worst* gag will break Paul up—he's on the *floor* laughing. There's a great willingness in him to play."

Finally, there's the racing. There's little doubt that the sport helps keep him young. "To be behind the wheel of a car doing over 100 mph is one of the most exhilarating things I know," he says. "Racing is a way of being a happy child again."

He also drives to test himself and to fight complacency. "You have to keep things off balance," he says, "or it's all over." Newman does little else besides race sports cars from April through October, and he's gotten very good at it—four times national champion in his class, and a billing by veteran driver Sam Posey as "one of the top endurance racers in the world."

According to Peter Slater of the Newman-Sharp Racing Team, Newman "has the mental outlook of a young, active person." Peter Bush says Newman "drives with the best of them. He's still got the fire.

There's a lot of talk of his retiring from racing—but I know for a fact he'll be back next year."

Taking the Years in Stride

So there it is. Paul Newman may be tired of his youthful image, but he seems to be doing all the right things to make sure it endures. He works out regularly and is careful about what he eats. He regularly tests himself and doesn't let boredom drag him down. He continues a love affair with his wife, and he has friends who are almost eerily devoted to him. And in what could be a crazy world of the rich and famous, he keeps things simple and sane: drives a Volkswagen Rabbit, does his own shopping, cooks his own food. As A. E. Hotchner told me, "He has a vital interest in life and surrounds himself with vital people."

Maybe the real secret behind Newman's graceful aging is his ambivalence about it. Beyond taking good care of himself, he refuses to be obsessed with aging gracefully. That's why he turns down interviews having to do with things like his appearance and takes on roles like Frank Galvin, the strung-out, over-the-hill lawyer in *The Verdict*. The primary factor in Newman being as young-acting as he is, says Don Kulowski, is that he doesn't dwell on his age.

—Hank Herman

PART 2

Healthy Eats

The High-Nutrition Superstars

Here are 25 of the finest foods for fitness. Find your best sources of protein, vitamins, minerals and fiber.

Food is fuel. It's simple, but it's true. Just as high-octane gas powers a car more efficiently, high-nutrient food delivers more energy to your body. If you want to be faster and stronger—if you want to last longer—you've got to use premium fuel.

Athletes have long tinkered with their diet to find the ideal foods for performance. And today, it's pretty widely agreed that a diet high in carbohydrates, modest in protein and—most important—low in fat delivers the most nutritional value. Even if you're not an athlete, your food choices make a big difference in how you feel. Eating right means feeling more alert and creative at work, less prone to afternoon blahs. "A couch potato and a marathon runner should eat the same foods," says Nancy Clark, registered dietitian and director of nutrition services at Sportsmedicine Brookline.

But getting your diet right isn't as easy as pulling up to the pump and pushing the "super" button. Not all carbohydrate sources are created equal. Some pack a more powerful punch than others, delivering more vitamins and minerals at a lower calorie cost. Likewise, some protein sources are richer and leaner than others.

While no single "perfect food" exists, many stand out as nutritional superstars. Following, in alphabetical order, is a guide to the good stuff: 25 first-class foods.

Bananas

The perfect portable snack. They're one of the richest sources of potassium, which may help regulate blood pressure, and good sources of fiber. Frozen banana chunks make a terrific guilt-free dessert. Bananas are also a natural antacid, according to a study published in *Lancet*.

One banana has 105 calories, 0.5 gram fat, 27 grams carbohydrate, 1.2 grams protein, 1 milligram sodium, 0 milligrams cholesterol, 2.2 grams fiber and 451 milligrams potassium.

Beans

An excellent source of fiber (important for keeping blood sugar and cholesterol levels under control). In fact, beans provide even more soluble fiber than oats. They're also high in protein and a good source of folate, a B vitamin important for building protein and red blood cells.

An average ½-cup serving has 112 calories, 0.4 gram fat, 21 grams carbohydrate, 7.5 grams protein, 1 milligram sodium, 0 milligrams cholesterol, 7.7 grams fiber, 304 milligrams potassium and 11 percent the U.S. Recommended Daily Allowance (USRDA) for folate.

Beef

Lots of people have been beef bashing lately, but truly lean beef is a great source of zinc, high-quality protein and iron. (The body absorbs the iron in meat more readily than the iron found in legumes, vegetables or breads.) Still, you need to be picky about the meat you buy. Choose only the leanest cuts, such as shank, round, flank and chuck. Look for "select" grades and trim fatty edges before cooking. Supermarkets now routinely offer "¼-inch trim" cuts, with the fat trimmed super close. You may also be able to find a new type of cut:

the "total trim," from which virtually all fat has been removed. These cuts are more expensive and are sold in smaller portions to help control serving sizes.

A 3-ounce serving of lean round steak has 163 calories, 5 grams fat, 0 grams carbohydrate, 27 grams protein, 56 milligrams sodium, 69 milligrams cholesterol, 0 grams fiber, 13 percent of the USRDA for iron, 32 percent of the USRDA for zinc and 41 percent of the USRDA for vitamin B_{12}.

Broccoli

A wonder food—one of the best nutrition bets around. Not only is broccoli high in fiber and vitamin C, but it also provides folate, calcium, magnesium and iron.

A 1-cup serving, cooked, has 46 calories, 0.4 gram fat, 9 grams carbohydrate, 5 grams protein, 16 milligrams sodium, 0 milligrams cholesterol, 4.8 grams fiber, 164 percent of the USRDA for vitamin C, 42 percent of the USRDA for vitamin A, 18 percent of the USRDA for calcium and 24 percent of the USRDA for folate.

Brown Rice

A good source of complex carbohydrates that provides twice as much fiber as white rice. Moreover, it beats white rice for almost every nutrient, including zinc, magnesium, protein, vitamin B_6, and selenium.

A ½-cup serving has 116 calories, 0.6 gram fat, 25 grams carbohydrate, 2.5 grams protein, 0 milligrams sodium, 0 milligrams cholesterol and 0.6 gram fiber.

Carrot Juice

Probably the most concentrated source of beta-carotene, which, in addition to its possible role as a cancer fighter, may play a key role in preventing the formation of cataracts later in life. Beta-carotene, a source of vitamin A, also may boost your immune system's ability to fight bacterial and viral infections, according to Joel Schwartz, Ph.D., associate professor at the Harvard School of Dental Medicine.

A ½-cup serving has 49 calories, 0.2 gram fat, 11 grams carbohydrate, 1 gram protein, 36 milligrams sodium, 0 milligrams cholesterol, 1.2 grams fiber and about 33 percent of the USRDA for vitamin A.

Chicken

Three ounces of skinless chicken breast has only 3 grams of fat and contains vitamin B_6, a nutrient important for metabolizing protein. Dark meat has more fat than white but also more B vitamins, iron, zinc and other nutrients. About skin: The usual advice is to cook the bird without it. (A thigh with skin can contain as much fat as beef.) But skin fat doesn't "migrate" into chicken meat, according to a letter in the *New England Journal of Medicine*. You may want to leave the skin on to keep the meat from drying out while cooking. Just don't give in to eating the crispy stuff later.

A 3-ounce breast with no skin, roasted, has 140 calories, 2.9 grams fat, 0 grams carbohydrate, 26 grams protein, 62 milligrams sodium, 0 grams fiber, 58 percent of the USRDA for niacin and 25 percent of the USRDA for vitamin B_6.

Corn

An often-overlooked source of fiber and carbohydrate. Sure, fresh corn tastes best, but frozen or canned alternatives are convenient ways to get additional fiber in your diet. Corn also has almost no fat.

A ½-cup serving has 67 calories, 0.6 gram fat, 17 grams carbohydrate, 2.5 grams protein, 4 milligrams sodium, 1.6 grams fiber and 17 micrograms folate.

Dried Fruit

Because most of the water has been removed, dried fruits are terrific concentrated sources of energy and good sources of iron—a mineral that helps prevent anemia. High in fructose, they also can be intensely sweet, making them great desserts or snacks—and they're fat-free. The following data are for dried apricots; pears, figs and raisins are similar.

A 3-ounce serving has 203 calories, 0.4 gram fat, 53 grams carbohydrate, 3.1 grams protein, 8.5 milligrams sodium, 0 milligrams cholesterol, 6.8 grams fiber, 22 percent of the USRDA for iron and 123 percent of the USRDA for vitamin A.

Fat-Free Yogurt

Among the few truly excellent sources of calcium—452 milligrams per 8-ounce carton—and riboflavin, yogurt's also a strong source of vitamin B_{12}. Use it to reduce fat in your diet: Substitute it for sour cream in casseroles or sauces; mix with herbs for vegetable dip; blend with fruit for a thick drink; stir into soups to make them creamy. Frozen, it's an excellent substitute for ice cream. To cut calories in half in flavored yogurts, choose brands artificially sweetened with aspartame (NutraSweet).

An 8-ounce serving (plain) has 127 calories, 0.4 gram fat, 17 grams carbohydrate, 13 grams protein, 174 milligrams sodium, 4 milligrams cholesterol, 0 grams fiber, 45 percent of the USRDA for calcium, 31 percent of the USRDA for riboflavin and 23 percent of the USRDA for vitamin B_{12}.

Fig Bars

A favorite among cyclists and runners because they pack a strong carbohydrate punch and are easy to eat during exercise. Much lower in fat than most treats, fig bars also supply a bit of fiber—not a lot, but more than most sweets.

Two bars have 106 calories, 1.9 grams fat, 21 grams carbohydrate, 1 gram protein, 90 milligrams sodium, 0 milligrams cholesterol and 5 grams fiber.

Grapes

Once thought to provide few significant nutrients. Now researchers from the U.S. Department of Agriculture say grapes are a good source of boron, a mineral believed to be important in building and maintaining healthy bones.

A ½-cup serving has 29 calories, 0.2 gram fat, 1 milligram sodium, 0 milligrams cholesterol and 0.3 gram fiber.

Kiwi

The odd little fruit in the fuzzy brown wrapper proves that good things come in small packages. Each kiwi provides 75 milligrams of vitamin C and 1.7 grams of fiber.

One kiwi has 46 calories, 0.3 gram fat, 11 grams carbohydrate, 0.8 gram protein, 4 milligrams sodium, 0 milligrams cholesterol, 1.7 grams fiber and 124 percent of the USRDA for vitamin C.

Lentils

Good sources of protein and complex carbohydrates. They also deliver a good amount of iron, particularly if you're limiting your intake of red meat. Lentils are easier to prepare than other legumes because you don't have to let them soak overnight before cooking. Great on their own, in soups or as an addition to ground meat.

A ½-cup serving has 105 calories, 0 grams fat, 20 grams carbohydrate, 8 grams protein, 30 milligrams sodium, 0 milligrams cholesterol, 5.2 grams fiber, 12 percent of the USRDA for iron, 7 percent of the USRDA for zinc and 9 percent of the USRDA for folate.

Low-Fat or Fat-Free Cheeses

These are great sources of calcium, but read nutrition labels carefully: Some of these cheeses aren't much lower in fat than regular counterparts, and they can be high in sodium. Choose one that contains 5 grams of fat or less per ounce.

A 1-ounce serving (Alpine Lace Colbi-Lo) has 85 calories, 5 grams fat, 7 grams protein, 85 milligrams sodium, 20 milligrams cholesterol and 35 percent of the USRDA for calcium.

Oatmeal

A good source of soluble fiber, and then some. In a study, adding 2 ounces of oatmeal a day to a low-fat diet significantly lowered subjects' blood cholesterol levels in about four weeks, according to registered dietitian and researcher Linda Van Horn, Ph.D., of Northwestern University Medical School in Chicago.

A ½-cup serving (regular) has 73 calories, 1.2 grams fat, 13 grams carbohydrate, 3 grams protein, 1 milligram sodium, 0 milligrams cholesterol and 2.7 grams fiber.

Orange Juice

Besides being an excellent source of vitamin C, one 6-ounce glass provides nearly as much potassium as a banana and about 23 percent of the USRDA for the sometimes hard-to-come-by B vitamin folate.

A 6-ounce serving has 76 calories, 0.3 gram fat, 18 grams carbo-hydrate, 1 gram protein, 1 milligram sodium, 0.1 gram fiber, 340 mil-ligrams potassium, 142 percent of the USRDA for vitamin C and 23 per-cent of the USRDA for folate.

Papaya

A treasure trove of nutrients. One-half of this exotic fruit provides almost as much potassium as a banana and more than 100 percent of the USRDA for vitamin C. It's also a good source of cancer-fighting beta-carotene.

One-half papaya has 59 calories, 0.2 gram fat, 15 grams carbohy-drate, 1 gram protein, 4 milligrams sodium, 0 milligrams cholesterol, 1.2 grams fiber, 395 milligrams potassium, 158 percent of the USRDA for vitamin C and about 62 percent of the USRDA for vitamin A.

Pasta

Loaded with complex carbohydrates for long-lasting energy, whether you're an athlete or a businessman. Enriched pasta also pro-vides iron and the important B vitamins thiamine, niacin and riboflavin.

A ½-cup serving has 77 calories, 0.3 gram fat, 28 grams carbo-hydrate, 5.3 grams protein, 0 milligrams cholesterol, 1 milligram sodium, 35 percent of the USRDA for thiamine, 15 percent of the USRDA for riboflavin, 15 percent of the USRDA for niacin and 10 per-cent of the USRDA for iron.

Potatoes

Probably one of the most underrated foods. Besides being a powerhouse of complex carbohydrates, a 6-ouncer also provides almost twice as much potassium as a banana, just over one-third of the USRDA for vitamin C and 66 percent of the USRDA for iron. It's also a good source of copper, which most people tend to be short on.

A 6-ounce potato with skin, baked, has 190 calories, 0.2 gram fat, 78 grams carbohydrate, 7 grams protein, 35 milligrams sodium, 0 mil-ligrams cholesterol, 4 grams fiber, 974 grams potassium, 38 percent of the USRDA for vitamin C, 66 percent of the USRDA for iron, 70 percent of the USRDA for copper and 56 percent of the USRDA for vitamin B_6.

Salmon

One of the richest sources of omega-3 fatty acids, which may provide some protection against heart disease. Eating salmon or other ocean fish such as mackerel, herring or tuna twice a week may be enough to reap the health benefits. Fish oil may also fight arthritis, alleviate psoriasis and reduce high blood pressure. Salmon is an excellent source of selenium, which the National Academy of Sciences says may play a role in cancer prevention.

A 3-ounce serving, cooked, has 157 calories, 6.4 grams fat, 0 grams carbohydrate, 23 grams protein, 50 milligrams sodium, 42 milligrams cholesterol, 0 grams fiber, 40 micrograms selenium, 42 percent of the USRDA for niacin and 35 percent of the USRDA for calcium. Most types of salmon provide about 1 gram of omega-3 fatty acids per 3-ounce serving.

Skim Milk

An excellent low-fat source of calcium and vitamin D—both important for maintaining healthy bones. Research suggests that you have less risk of developing colon cancer with high blood levels of vitamin D than with low levels. But don't turn to supplements for vitamin D: Large amounts can be toxic.

An 8-ounce serving has 80 calories, 0.4 gram fat, 11 grams carbohydrate, 8 grams protein, 4 milligrams cholesterol, 117 milligrams sodium, 0 grams fiber, 24 percent of the USRDA for vitamin D and 28 percent of the USRDA for calcium.

Strawberries

Sweet, delicious strawberries are excellent sources of vitamin C and fiber. They also contain ellagic acid, which may prove important in cancer prevention, according to researcher Gary Stoner, Ph.D., director of experimental pathology at the Medical College of Ohio.

A 1-cup serving has 45 calories, 0.6 gram fat, 11 grams carbohydrate, 1 gram protein, 2 milligrams sodium, 0 milligrams cholesterol, 2.2 grams fiber and 141 percent of the USRDA for vitamin C.

Water

The most critical nutrient in your body, it's needed for just about everything that happens, and you lose it fast: at least 2 cups daily just exhaling; 10 cups through normal waste and body cooling; 1 to 2 quarts per hour running, biking or working out. Eight glasses a day is enough for sedentary folks, but if you're physically active, you need more. Drink 8 to 20 ounces of water about 15 minutes before working out. If you run, drink at least 2 cups of water for every pound you lose on your course.

Whole-Grain Cereals

Besides providing lots of complex carbohydrates, they're a great way to get fiber in your diet—a prevention measure that the National Cancer Institute strongly recommends. What's more, research suggests that eating a high-fiber cereal at breakfast may curb your appetite at lunch. Read the labels: A cereal should contain at least 5 grams of fiber and no more than 1 or 2 grams of fat per serving. Some cereals that trumpet themselves as being high in fiber actually provide insignificant amounts and may have as much fat per serving as a pat of butter. Don't worry too much about the sugar content. Actually, a bowl of low-fat but sugary cereal with skim milk is a much better antidote to a sweet tooth than a bowl of ice cream or a hunk of fat-laden cake.

—Densie Webb, Ph.D.

Eat to Compete

A few simple nutritional guidelines can boost any athlete's performance. Follow these six rules, and you may find yourself breaking new ground.

To the athlete, food can be a friend or a foe. What you eat today will bear on how well you perform tomorrow and the next day. Even the best diet isn't a substitute for talent and training, but the right foods will help you make the most of what you've got.

Unfortunately, good intentions tend to break down at moments of crisis. As you stare at the menu in a restaurant, you can't remember

---

Heavy Hitters

The top ten sources of protein and carbohydrates:

PROTEIN		CARBOHYDRATES	
Lean meats	Yogurt	Potatoes	Lentils
Poultry	Nuts	Breads	Cereals
Fish	Beans	Rice	Beans
Tofu	Skim milk	Pasta	Corn
Cheese	Lentils	Fruits	Peas

---

what's better for you than what else, let alone why. At times like these, the whole business of trying to eat right begins to seem like an abstract, obscure nuisance. If everyone else at the table orders steak with béarnaise sauce, "Me, too" is simpler than trying to mentally call up charts and graphs of calories and fat grams.

Forget trying to grasp and apply the complicated chemistry of metabolism, and instead memorize these six rules. If you can remember to use them, you'll be able to choose the right foods to eat, even under difficult circumstances.

Rule 1: Eat protein for strength, carbohydrates for endurance. The basic concept behind your food choices is that food is fuel. An athlete eats to build strength and endurance. Eat high-protein foods for more power, complex carbohydrates for stamina. Quality protein comes from meats and fish, complex carbohydrates from plants. Eat them both.

Rule 2: Two-thirds carbohydrates, one-third protein. Now for the technical stuff. Rule 2 is actually the rule of threes. Imagine that your plate is divided into three equal areas. By volume, two-thirds of your plate should be covered by complex carbohydrates, one-third by your protein item. Of course, you should also eat your vegetables, but you and your mom can discuss that elsewhere.

Rule 3: Eat white. Life is difficult enough without having to make technical food choices at socially sensitive moments, so memorize Rule 3 and eat foods that are white or tan. With minimal rational thought, this rule will result in a diet of potatoes, brown rice, grains, pasta and cereals (all complex carbohydrates), as well as fish and chicken. But forget cream sauces. The chef is trying to kill you.

Rule 4: In near-terminal fatigue, remember potatoes. The fourth rule is for use when you're too tired to think, let alone cook: Nuke a spud. A baked potato can be produced in five minutes in your microwave. Top it with salsa, vegetarian chili, or low-fat yogurt. The potato is an athlete's best friend, chock-full of complex carbohydrates, cheap, quick and easy to cook. If you don't sabotage its innocence with butter and sour cream, a potato contains no fat. While the potato cooks, make yourself a salad and you'll have a meal that provides you with both the building blocks of athletic excellence and the Recommended Dietary Allowance (RDA) of moral superiority.

Rule 5: Put light food on a dark plate for visual relief. The above dietary plan has one drawback: It makes for a dull meal and a boring lifestyle, which leads us to Rule 5. A gleaming black plate will make your white dinner look snazzy, even art deco, sort of. Add a few green vegetables ornamentally, for your mother's sake.

Rule 6: Give it a rest sometimes. When your tolerance for eating right flags, give it a break. A diet is not a religion. Know the rules and follow them when you can, but don't be too hard on yourself if you feel like blowing it all off once in a while.

See you at the finish line.

—Anne Robinson

Healthy Snacks for Men on the Run

Healthy meals needn't take hours to prepare. Got a few minutes for some helpful pointers?

When the American Dietetic Association polled men, 82 percent of them said they were concerned about their nutrition. Concern, however, doesn't always translate into actually doing something. Only about one-half of those surveyed said they were making changes in their diet as a result of their concerns.

Why the gap between intention and action? Probably because while many of us want to take better care of ourselves, we can't make a full-time job out of it. (One of those is quite enough, thank you.) If it's going to be a lot of hassle and bother, we'll just have to get around to it later. *Much* later.

Procrastinate no more. Here are 25 quick and simple ways you can get a start toward a more healthful diet.

Breakfast

1. Start your morning with a heaping bowl of cereal and you'll likely eat less fat and cholesterol throughout the day—even compared with those who eat something else for breakfast, according to research at St. Joseph's University. High-fiber cereals—ones that contain at least 4 grams of fiber per serving—are better for you, but even sugar-laden kiddie cereals appear to have this fat-curbing effect.

2. Soften butter or margarine at room temperature. Chances are you'll spread your bread with one-quarter of the fat and calories you do when you put it down cold. If you forget, use the microwave.

3. Spread your toast or bagel with fruit preserves or jam, which are fat-free, instead of butter or margarine. You'll save about 4 grams of fat for every pat you don't use.

4. Although whole milk contains only 3.3 percent fat, that measurement is by weight. The true, meaningful measurement of fat is actually percentage of calories from fat, and *49 percent* of the calories in whole milk come from fat. Low-fat, or 2 percent, milk isn't much better: Fully 35 percent of its calories come from saturated fat. But skim milk gets only 5 percent of its calories from fat.

In coffee, evaporated canned skim milk makes a decent substitute for half-and-half.

5. Fresh orange juice has more vitamin C than orange juice made from frozen concentrate. Many supermarkets and delis now sell fresh-squeezed, but don't buy more than you can use in four days, since juice begins to lose its vitamin C after it's been opened.

6. Some men just can't face food in the morning. If you're one of them, a good-quality liquid instant breakfast is better than noth-ing. Look for a product that's low in sugar and that provides one-third of the Recommended Dietary Allowances (RDAs) of vitamins and minerals.

7. If you take vitamin supplements in the morning, you should know how to get the most out of them. Fat-soluble vitamins (A, D and E) are absorbed best when taken with foods that contain fat. Take them with a glass of milk. Water-soluble vitamins (C and the Bs) should be taken either during a meal or about a half hour before or after eating. Vitamin C should be taken in a few small doses during the day rather than in one big dose.

Lunch

8. Try canned pink salmon in sandwiches. Salmon is high in potassium and calcium and tastes great with cheese and vegetables. Or prepare a low-fat version of tuna salad by combining a can of drained water-packed tuna with a tablespoon of red wine vinegar and chopped onions to taste.

9. Turn a can of low-sodium broth (beef or chicken) into a quick, healthy meal by adding fresh or frozen vegetables, cooked chicken chunks or diced tofu, fresh or dried herbs and a little sherry or freshly grated ginger and/or hot pepper sauce.

To defat the broth, refrigerate it for a few hours, then skim off all the fat that congeals on the top.

10. Deli sandwiches with all the trimmings aren't the worst things to have for lunch—particularly if you do without the fatty sauces and avoid salt- and smoke-cured meats like bologna, ham and salami. A case in point: Without sauce, lean roast beef sandwiches are fine.

11. Salad bars can provide the fixings for a nutritious, filling and low-calorie lunch—or a fat-laden dietary disaster. Here's how to make smart choices:

• Ignore the iceberg lettuce in favor of spinach or romaine or leaf lettuce. They contain more vitamin A and calcium.

• Dip deep into the beans, peas, beets, sliced mushrooms, cucumbers, tomatoes, green peppers, grated carrots, broccoli and cauliflower. One-half cup of peas, beans and broccoli gives you over 2 grams of fiber.

• Go easy on the grated cheese.

• If you want a garnish of meat, pick the shrimp, chicken or turkey. Only 20 percent of their calories come from fat.

• Skip the ham, chopped eggs, croutons, bacon bits and fried noodles and the salads made with mayonnaise.

• Use no more than 1 tablespoon of dressing, even if there is reduced-calorie available. (The round dippers on most salad bars are the equivalent of 2 tablespoons.)

12. You can make a baked potato flavorful with a few drops of extra-virgin olive oil, soy sauce or Worcestershire sauce, or an herb-and-spice blend. Try this: Mash tofu with a little low-fat mayonnaise, then add curry and herb seasonings to taste.

Dinner

13. Start with a high-carbohydrate food, such as a pasta appetizer, bread without butter or a bean or noodle soup. Studies show that doing so will lessen your appetite.

14. Oven-fried chicken tastes great—without a trace of added fat. Rub skinless chicken pieces with prepared mustard, then coat them with yellow cornmeal. Bake at 450°F for 15 minutes, then lower the temperature to 350°F and bake another 20 minutes or until cooked through.

15. Fish is good food, low in saturated fat and rich in artery-protecting omega-3's. And shellfish lovers should take note that clams, mussels, oysters and crabs, once suspected of harboring too much cholesterol, have now been put in the clear. But two others, shrimp and squid, still deliver astoundingly high amounts of cholesterol and should be eaten in moderation.

16. We have no beef with beef, as long as it's eaten in moderation. To make sure you get the leanest meat, check the grade. "Prime" and "choice" cuts are the highest in cholesterol. What makes them so tender and juicy is fat. As you descend the meat industry's rating chart, you ascend in health. The "good" and "select" cuts have less fat, fewer calories and less cholesterol.

Grill your steaks or cook them on a rack or in a slotted pan to let some of the remaining fat drip away. Never rub a steak with oil before cooking it; that will seal in most of the fat.

17. Make your own pizza dough (or buy it ready-made), but instead of the usual toppings, try vegetables such as carrots, onions, peppers and broccoli, either stir-fried in a bit of oil or (better yet) steamed. Top with part-skim mozzarella and bake as usual. Instead of pepperoni, sprinkle on some ground turkey or turkey sausage that you've taken out of its casing.

18. For a fast, nutritious, low-calorie dessert, microwave an apple. Peel the top third to prevent the insides from bursting as the heat expands them. Cover the apple and cook on full power for 3 minutes. Top with low-fat or nonfat yogurt flavored with maple syrup and cinnamon.

Snacks

19. A frozen juice bar (almost no fat) is a much more healthful cool snack option than an ice-cream bar (15 to 25 grams of fat). If you must have something cold and creamy, have a pudding pop (about 2 grams of fat).

20. Never eat foods out of their original containers. How many times have you dipped into a pint of ice cream with the intention of having "just a tad," only to find yourself staring at the bottom of the container 15 minutes later? You're much less likely to do that if you dish out the food in a measured portion.

21. Before giving in to that craving for a piece of candy, try brushing your teeth. The sweetness of the toothpaste may take your craving away, and the flavor it leaves in your mouth may make you rethink that handful of jelly beans.

22. Read food labels for clues on sugar content. If the name sugar, sucrose, glucose, maltose, dextrose, lactose, fructose, corn syrup or any other syrup appears first or near the top of the list, there is a large amount of sugar in that product.

23. Choose pretzels over potato chips or prepackaged popcorn. Pretzels contain about 1 gram of fat per ounce; many chips have ten times that much.

24. An apple a day keeps the droopiness away, suggest scientists at the federal government's Human Nutrition Research Center in Grand Forks, North Dakota. They find that boron-rich foods improve motor skills and boost alertness. Apples and other noncitrus foods such as broccoli, peas, beans and cabbage are good sources of boron, which also helps the body better retain calcium.

Apples are also good for your teeth. They crunch among the teeth's spaces, dislodging the cavity creators and stimulating saliva flow to counteract plaque, says Elaine M. Parker, former assistant professor of dental hygiene at the University of Maryland.

25. In general, the more the cookie crumbles, the better it is for you. Softer-textured cookies tend to have a higher fat content, with one exception being fig bars. Harder cookies like gingersnaps and vanilla wafers have about one-half the fat of their soft cousins.

Better yet, skip fat-laden cookies and munch on crackers instead. Although some crackers still contain lard, the total amount of fat per serving is much less than the amount in cookies. In general, figure four crackers are equivalent in fat to one cookie.

—Nick Barton

Nine Nutrients for Men

Men need more of just about every essential nutrient than women do. Here are the nine most important vitamins and minerals that every man should know about.

Which vitamins do you need most, and how much do you need? *Men's Health* went to the experts for the answers. But first, an interesting footnote: Men and women have differing nutritional needs. In fact, the U.S. Food and Drug Administration puts out separate men's and women's lists of Recommended Dietary Allowances (RDAs) for vitamins and minerals. And men need more of just about every essential nutrient than women do. Why? Quite simply, because we're bigger. We have more muscle and burn more calories than women do. And those of us who are fit and active, in particular, need higher quantities of certain key nutrients.

Further, getting enough of the right vitamins and minerals can help us fight problems we men are at especially high risk for, such as elevated cholesterol, hypertension, coronary heart disease, stroke, certain cancers and kidney stones.

Here, in alphabetical order, are the nine nutrients men need most.

Chromium

This vital mineral can cut cholesterol, boost endurance in athletes and help bodybuilders gain muscle and lose fat. The average man needs at least 50 micrograms of chromium a day, but active men should get 100 to 200 micrograms, according to Richard Anderson, Ph.D., of the U.S. Department of Agriculture Human Nutrition Research Center. "You'll have a hard time getting this much from foods," he says. Your best source is a multivitamin/mineral complex that includes chromium. Next best is one or two chromium-fortified tablets of brewer's yeast daily.

Fiber

Technically, fiber's not a nutrient, since it passes through the body undigested. But eating fiber substantially reduces cholesterol and may help lower blood pressure. A high-fiber diet may lower your risk of colon cancer (the third most common kind for men) and can control sugar levels in diabetics. Fiber may even help you lose weight by filling you up without a lot of calories. Two medium-size apples will give you 14 of the recommended 18 to 35 daily grams of dietary fiber you need. You also get fiber from whole-grain breads and breakfast cereals, brown rice, strawberries, pears and vegetables, especially ones with edible stalks and stems such as broccoli and carrots.

Magnesium

This mineral plays a key role in regulating the heartbeat—studies show that getting enough may protect men against heart disease as well as bring down high blood pressure. Magnesium also boosts fertility by making sperm more vigorous. You'll get about two-thirds of your daily requirement of magnesium from a breakfast of two cups of shredded wheat, skim milk and a banana. Baked potatoes, beans, nuts, oatmeal, peanut butter, whole-wheat spaghetti, leafy vegetables and seafood are also magnesium rich.

Vitamin A

Studies find vitamin A can have significant immunity-boosting and anticancer effects. And, yes, just as your mother told you, it helps maintain good vision. A ½-cup serving of steamed carrots supplies almost four times a man's daily recommended intake of 1,000 milligrams. Other good sources are liver, dairy products, fish, tomatoes, apricots and cantaloupe. Vitamin A is easy to get from your diet and extremely toxic in high doses, so experts recommend avoiding supplements.

Vitamin B₆

This necessary nutrient is a powerful immune booster, and some studies suggest it may prevent skin and bladder cancer. Additionally, B_6 protects against the formation of kidney stones (a problem that afflicts twice as many men as women) and can help prevent restless sleep. You need only 2 milligrams of vitamin B_6 daily—about the amount in two large bananas. Active men need a few milligrams more, since it's burned up during exercise, says Paula Trumbo, Ph.D., assistant professor of nutritional biochemistry at Purdue University. Other dietary sources include chicken and fish, liver, potatoes, avocados and sunflower seeds. High doses of B_6 supplements can be toxic over time, so experts recommend taking no more than 50 milligrams a day.

Vitamin C

It boosts immunity; may help prevent cancer, heart disease and stroke; promotes healthy gums and teeth; prevents cataracts; hastens wound healing; counteracts asthma; and may help overcome infertility in men. Keeping your body well supplied with vitamin C may also slow the aging process. Broccoli, cantaloupe, green peppers and grapefruit juice are good dietary sources, but taking supplements won't harm you, as this vitamin's not toxic in high doses. Researcher Earl Dawson, Ph.D., of the University of Texas Medical Branch, says 200 to 300 milligrams a day should be adequate. Many researchers think you'll shortchange yourself on vitamin C with the RDA of 60 milligrams (the amount in ½ cup of fresh orange juice), particularly when it comes to warding off the common cold, the most well known of C's many benefits.

If you smoke, you probably need extra vitamin C. Smokers have lower levels of the vitamin in their blood. No one knows why, but the implication is that their bodies need more C and thus are using more.

Vitamin E

Studies show vitamin E lowers cholesterol, prevents buildup of artery-clogging plaque, boosts immunity, cleanses the body of pollutants and prevents cataracts. There's lots of vitamin E in almonds, peanuts and pecans, but it's hard to get enough of this nutrient from your diet. Fortunately, supplements are safe in doses much higher than the 10-milligram RDA. Biochemist Max Horwitt, Ph.D., of the St. Louis University School of Medicine, takes 269 milligrams daily and considers that amount safe.

Water

It's the most essential of all nutrients, especially if you're muscular: Muscle contains almost three times more water than fat. (The average man's body is 40 percent muscle, while the average woman's is 23 percent.) Water lubricates joints, regulates temperature and provides the body with minerals and essential fluids. The average man should get at least two quarts a day, or about eight glasses. "If you're physically active, you easily could need to double that," says Georgia Kostas, a registered dietitian and director of nutrition at the Cooper Clinic. You also get water from food: Bread is about 36 percent water; a potato, 80 percent.

Zinc

Getting enough zinc ensures that your sex drive, potency and fertility stay in shape. Zinc has been used experimentally to treat impotence, and it has a profound influence on the body's ability to heal wounds and resist disease. Men tend to get only about two-thirds the RDA of 15 milligrams, particularly if we're active. That's because when men sweat, we lose more zinc than women. One four-ounce helping of lean beef provides almost half the daily zinc needs. Other good sources are turkey, seafood, cereals and beans. Too much zinc can hinder the work of other minerals, so experts recommend taking no more than one 15-milligram supplement a day.

—Richard Laliberte

Designated Eaters

Looking for healthful substitutes for high-fat, high-calorie and low-fiber foods? Here are some smart swaps to get you on the healthy track.

When it comes to eating healthier, our motto is "Switch, don't fight." Don't do battle with your urges for satisfying foods in a quest for less fat and calories and more fiber; just switch to equally satisfying but more healthful alternatives.

An example: On the gratification scale, a roast beef sandwich with cheese comes close to a large cheeseburger, but the roast beef contains 43 percent less fat and 101 fewer calories. Not a bad deal.

If you find that one of these swaps doesn't immediately ring the same bells as its less healthy cousin, give it another chance. It often takes a little time for your brain's "pleasure centers" to adapt to something slightly different.

Instead of . . .	Try . . .	Benefit
Salted peanuts	Pretzels	91% less fat
Potato chips	Popcorn, air-popped	96% less fat
Saltines	Animal crackers	22% less fat
Chocolate chip cookies	Fig bars	80% less fat
Caramels	Raisins	96% less fat
Pecan pie	Chocolate cake w/icing	32% less fat
Chocolate cake w/icing	Apple pie	28% less fat
Eclairs w/custard filling and chocolate icing	Angel food cake w/chocolate syrup	96% less fat
Glazed doughnuts	Blueberry muffins	59% less fat
Granola cereal	Raisin bran	89% less fat
Peanut butter on bagel	Strawberry jam on bagel	99% less fat
Italian roll	Whole-wheat bread	87% more fiber
Regular mayonnaise on burger	Barbecue sauce on burger	84% less fat

(continued)

Instead of . . .	Try . . .	Benefit
Large cheeseburger	Roast beef sandwich w/cheese	101 fewer calories
Beef bologna	Turkey bologna	47% less fat
Sandwich w/cold cuts	Sandwich w/roast beef	27% less fat
Pepperoni pizza	Cheese pizza	48% less fat
Bean-and-meat burrito	Bean burrito	19% less fat
Macaroni and cheese	Spaghetti in tomato sauce w/cheese	170 fewer calories/cup
Prime rib, roasted	Sirloin, broiled	67% less fat
Chicken drumsticks, roasted	Chicken breasts, roasted	30% less fat
Steamed salmon	Baked cod	89% less fat
Lamb shoulder	Leg of lamb	28% less fat
Chocolate milk, whole	Chocolate milk, 1%	71% less fat
Half-and-half in coffee	Condensed skim milk in coffee	98% less fat

Note: Except where indicated, this chart compares 100-gram portions of each food.

—*Mary Brophy*

Power Eating

We asked the medical experts to design an eating plan for total health. They came up with a dozen steps to peak nutrition.

There is certainly no shortage of self-proclaimed nutrition "experts" out there, from fitness gurus who make millions selling worthless supplement powders and pills to next-door neighbors who claim that eating white bread will send you to an early grave.

Who has the time to weigh all the contradictory advice, much less judge the validity of its source? Not you. And anyway, that's why you read books like this one.

To get straight answers for our readers, *Men's Health* surveyed 300 of the nation's top nutrition experts—not the self-appointed kind, but the ones doing important research at major hospitals and universities. Medical Consensus Surveys, a research arm of Rodale Press, asked the experts to rate 44 nutritional actions (all purported to benefit health) as follows: Extremely Important, Very Important, Important, Not Important or Probably Worthless.

What we were after was a list of priorities, a simple guide to making smart nutritional choices. For example, should you put a lot of energy into reducing the amount of cholesterol in your diet? The amount of salt? Or is it more important to avoid pesticides, irradiated food or alcohol?

The nutritionists' responses were then compiled and statistically weighted to create a list of dietary priorities that's both clear and practical. "We could easily have an enormous advance in the health of America if we could simply follow these guidelines," says George L. Blackburn, M.D., Ph.D., chief of the Nutrition/Metabolism Laboratory at New England Deaconess Hospital in Boston.

Here, in order of importance, are the nutritional steps most vital to your healthy diet, and the stuff that's not worth worrying about.

Get the Fat Out

The experts were almost unanimous in putting weight control at the top of the list—97 percent of them gave it high priority.

"If everybody in the United States maintained their ideal weight, the incidence of Type-II diabetes would be greatly reduced, hypertension would be much less common and so would coronary disease," says Meir Stampfer, M.D., associate professor of epidemiology at Harvard School of Public Health.

Nearly 24 percent of American men are overweight for their age and build, which makes obesity one of the country's biggest health problems.

How do the experts recommend we lose weight? Seventy-five percent said that cutting calories is extremely important or very important; 70 percent said the same about controlling fat intake. The two go hand in hand: If you cut calories, you'll cut fat. The number of calories you eat ultimately determines how much you'll weigh, but reducing fat is important for other reasons: It slashes the risk of heart disease by keeping arteries from choking with plaque, and it may reduce the risk of some forms of cancer.

Eat and Run

Strictly speaking, exercise isn't a nutritional habit, but we included it in our survey because physical activity has a direct bearing on how much we eat and on what happens to food once we've taken it in. The experts affirmed this view, and then some. Eighty-four percent gave high priority to exercising more. "It's hard to reduce your weight by controlling calories alone," says Dr. Stampfer. "If you exercise as well, you're more likely to be able to maintain the weight loss in the long run."

Exercise boosts your metabolism, allowing you to eat more without putting on more pounds. It also helps relieve stress and keep your heart, bones and circulatory system in top form.

Most people can fill their exercise quota with 20 minutes of brisk walking three times a week. Adding a regimen of resistance weight training fires up your metabolism to its calorie-burning peak.

Don't Like It, Don't Eat It

Giving up all your favorite foods and switching to a very healthy but very boring diet won't work. Kelly Brownell, Ph.D., professor of psychology at Yale University and a top obesity researcher, says he and others have studied dieters and found that the most punishing methods inevitably fail.

Nobody is going to eat food they don't enjoy for very long. If you want to eat healthy, you have to either find low-fat prepared foods that taste great or learn to cook your own.

Keep It Balanced but Lean

You've heard the old nutritionist's creed: Balance your diet among the four food groups and make sure you get the Recommended Dietary Allowance (RDA) of vitamins and minerals. These concepts are certainly not passé; roughly 90 percent of those surveyed said they're still high priority. Yet those notions now clearly take a backseat to cutting fat and controlling weight.

The weakness of the four-food-groups approach is that it doesn't provide enough guidance to prevent you from eating too much fat and amassing too much of it on your body.

If you make fat-fighting your number one priority, however, it quite naturally leads you toward fulfilling those other guidelines. "If you phase out the high-calorie, high-fat foods in your diet, you're going to have to replace them with something low-fat—cereals, fruits and vegetables," says Dr. Blackburn. An emphasis on those foods moves you closer to meeting your RDA for vitamins and minerals. It can also move you closer to balancing your diet, which for most Americans is overladen with high-fat meat and dairy products.

Don't Sweat the Technicalities

If you've never been able to keep straight the difference between saturated, unsaturated, monounsaturated and polyunsaturated fats, here's good news: You don't have to. The trendy notion that you should trade saturated fats for heart-smarter monounsaturated and polyunsaturated ones is "putting the cart before the horse," according to Dr. Blackburn. Most of the foods that are highest in total fat—ice cream, cheeseburgers and doughnuts, for example—are also highest in saturated fat. So if you simply cut down on all fatty foods, you'll cut down on saturated fat as well.

How much fat should you eat? The nutritionists advise following the American Heart Association's recommendation that total dietary fat comprise no more than 30 percent of calories.

Let Cholesterol Take Care of Itself

Cutting cholesterol scored surprisingly low. Only 14 percent of the experts rated it extremely important. It's not that cholesterol is insignificant, but, again, if you follow the priorities outlined above, you'll have already taken care of it. Those polled felt that excessive concern about this issue to the exclusion of all others could lead you to eat foods that are low in cholesterol but still dangerously high in fat. For example, potato chips fried in vegetable oil contain no cholesterol, but 72 percent of their calories are from fat.

Don't Fear Saying "Cheers"

The nation's top nutritionists plainly don't support prohibition. But they're staunch believers in moderation when it comes to alcohol. "There's no evidence, unless you are driving, that drinking alcohol in limited quantities is bad for you," says Judith S. Stern, Sc.D., a registered dietitian and professor of nutrition at the University of California, Davis. Alcohol in excess (more than two drinks per day) is another story: It'll destroy livers as well as lives.

Practice Safe Eating

While many people are worried about pesticides on fruits and vegetables, the experts rated it 34 out of 44 on their list of priorities.

More than three-quarters of the nutritionists thought it wise to avoid raw foods, particularly eggs, meat and seafood. Raw eggs and chicken can harbor salmonella bacteria, a common cause of food poisoning. Raw seafood can harbor viruses or parasites. Buy only from a reputable dealer or avoid raw seafood altogether.

Get More Fiber

Insoluble or soluble? It doesn't matter how you get your fiber. What's important is just that you do get it. "People eat so little fiber, we'll take anything," says Dr. Blackburn. "Whatever you can find— some peas in your stew—put them in!"

A high-fiber diet fills you up without filling you out, keeps you regular, helps lower your cholesterol level and may help reduce the risk of colon cancer. The nutritionists advocate getting at least 20 grams per day. A breakfast of oatmeal, whole-wheat toast, a pear and a banana would give you more than half that amount. The highest-fiber foods are fruits, vegetables, whole grains and legumes.

More Surf, Less Turf

Fish is lower in saturated fat than meat, and the oil in fish—especially cold-water varieties such as salmon and mackerel—helps your cardiovascular system by keeping blood from clotting and preventing hardening of the arteries. If you do eat meat, the experts recommend limiting portions to three or four ounces, choosing lean cuts such as flank steak and using low-fat cooking methods such as broiling and braising.

Avoid Fads

Many nutrition hazards you read or hear about on the 11 o'clock news aren't worth paying attention to, according to our experts. For example, avoiding trans-fatty acids (found in stick margarine) and trop-

FOOD FACTS, FOOD FADS

The numbers in the following table indicate how valuable *Men's Health*'s 300-plus experts think these actions are for a healthy diet. The higher the number, the greater its importance.

Score	Action
	HIGH PRIORITY
79	Control calories to control weight
76	Reduce all dietary fats
71	Increase physical activity
71	Enjoy your food
70	Eat a balanced diet
69	Get the RDAs of vitamins and minerals
65	Reduce saturated fats
65	Limit alcohol intake
63	Avoid raw eggs, meat and seafood
62	Boost fiber to 20 grams per day
61	Eat fish instead of meat
	LOW PRIORITY
16	Make breakfast the biggest meal of the day
14	Avoid irradiated foods
13	Avoid charred or blackened foods

ical oils drew only moderate priority ratings from the nutrition authorities, despite their getting big play in the news. Again, it's much more important to lower *total* fat intake.

The experts also said most of us need not worry about sugar. It's a problem for people who are obese (it's got lots of calories but little nutrition) or diabetic (they can't metabolize it properly). For the rest of us, though, avoiding sugar is only of moderate importance.

Rated lowest of all was avoiding irradiated foods—68 percent of respondents put this among the probably worthless, right down there with avoiding charred or blackened foods. Neither appears to pose any significant health risk.

Stop Watching the Clock

Our experts gave only a moderate priority rating to avoiding snacks and eating three square meals a day. It seems the nutrition masters are trying to tell us something: What you eat is much more important than how or when you eat.

—Susan Zarrow

It's the Better Thing to Do

Oat bran may get all the press coverage, but psyllium is the superstar when it comes to lowering your cholesterol.

Get me Hollywood. Time for *Mary Poppins II*. We get Julie Andrews. She sings. But forget that spoonful of sugar stuff. Times change. This time it's: "A spoonful of psyllium helps the cholesterol go down. . . ." Think of the commercial tie-ins. Memo to Madison Avenue: We'll blow Wilford Brimley right off the tube. . . .

Okay, so we're making lowering cholesterol sound suspiciously easy. But we figure anything worth doing is worth doing the easy way, and, besides, this psyllium stuff really seems to work.

Oat bran and psyllium are both sources of soluble fiber, which helps lower cholesterol. Lately, studies have questioned whether oat bran's effect comes from the fiber itself, or from the fact that an oat-bran muffin simply fills you up, making you less likely to tackle an Egg McMuffin afterward. Either way, psyllium is a much better source of soluble fiber than oat bran.

Psyllium is a grain grown in India and the Mediterranean, and it happens to be nature's all-time great source of soluble fiber. It takes about eight teaspoons of oat bran (or about 1½ bowls of oatmeal) to match the amount of soluble fiber in a single teaspoon of psyllium. Of course, if you're a label reader, none of this is news to you; psyllium is used in bulk-forming laxatives (such as Metamucil and Fiberall), and recently it's been added to some breakfast cereals.

Just What the Doctor Ordered

All of which seem to be just what the doctors are ordering. "We encourage people to use psyllium in addition to changing their diet," says Donald Smith, M.D., a lipids and metabolism researcher at the Mount Sinai Medical Center in New York. "Soluble fiber really does reduce the harmful form of cholesterol, whether you get the fiber from fruit, vegetables, beans, grains or psyllium."

In one study, men who ate a typical American diet took a teaspoon of psyllium three times a day for eight weeks and dropped their levels of harmful cholesterol by 20 percent. (Every 1 percent decrease in cholesterol means a 2 percent decrease in the incidence of heart attacks.) In another study, harmful cholesterol decreased an additional 8 percent among men who ate a low-fat diet plus psyllium, as compared with those who just dieted.

Psyllium may also help you lose weight, according to George L. Blackburn, M.D., Ph.D., chief of the Nutrition/Metabolism Laboratory at New England Deaconess Hospital in Boston. High-fiber foods take longer to digest, so your stomach feels full longer and you eat less.

Just don't take that as license to eat anything you want as long as you follow it with a few teaspoons of fiber. "There's a rumor going around that you can lose weight on ice cream and candy bars as long as you send them down the hatch with some fiber," says Dr. Blackburn. "The claim is that the fiber will escort a large portion of the calories out the back door. That's a wild exaggeration."

When you're ready to lower your cholesterol, the first step is to switch to a low-fat diet and to include some oat bran in your meals. Then, says Peter Kwiterovich, Jr., M.D., author of *Beyond Cholesterol: The Johns Hopkins Complete Guide for Avoiding Heart Disease,* if your cholesterol level is still borderline high (200 to 240) or high (over 240), ask your doctor if you should be taking one teaspoon of powdered psyllium three times a day to achieve an additional reduction. Metamucil is probably the best-known psyllium product, but there are dozens of brands of psyllium in powdered and tablet form at pharmacies and health-food stores. Dr. Smith of Mount Sinai recommends stirring powdered psyllium into an eight-ounce glass of water before meals.

If you begin your day with a high-fiber breakfast (a one-ounce serving of Kellogg's Heartwise cereal, which contains psyllium, gives you close to a teaspoon of soluble fiber), you can skip your morning teaspoon of psyllium and take only two teaspoons later.

Don't Overdo It

Just don't overdo it, warns Dr. Blackburn. More fiber is not necessarily better, and too much can cause stomach upset, gas and diarrhea.

And what if you have no reason to assume you're among the unlucky one in five American men with a cholesterol level in the risky zones above 200?

"I'd recommend taking psyllium anyway," says Larry Bell, M.D., of the University of Minnesota, whose psyllium research appeared in the *Journal of the American Medical Association*. "Whether it lowers your cholesterol or not, many health groups recommend that we get more fiber in our diets."

Remember, the longer your cholesterol stays elevated, the greater your danger of heart disease. A diet that's low in fat and high in soluble fiber, including psyllium, is a way to eat smart and protect your heart.

—*Douglas Carpenter*

PART 3

Men at Ease

The Balanced Life

Every man—including you—needs a minimum daily dose of fun. Laughs may be essential to good health.

To be a man of robust health, be a man of many pleasures, advises preventive-medicine specialist and author David Sobel, M.D. Having fun, feeling satisfied, loving someone or finding something deeply agreeable to spend some time on, he says, produces healthy states in your brain and body. He points to evidence that shows that cultivating the simple joys of daily life can boost your immunity, lower your blood pressure, help ward off heart disease, relieve pain and maybe even guard against certain types of cancer. "Pleasure is a prescription for well-being that's filled in the pharmacy of the brain," writes Dr. Sobel, coauthor of the book *Healthy Pleasures. Men's Health* talked with him about the role of fun and games in our health.

Q. You begin your book by explaining the Pleasure Principle. Can you sum that up?

A. I've spent the past 20 years looking at what makes people healthy. It turns out that the hardiest, most vital people tend to be pleasure-loving, pleasure-seeking, pleasure-creating people. They enjoy many small daily pleasures, from the sensual to the intellectual to helping others. And this theme of pleasure seems to run through their lives. They *expect* each day to feel good.

This led us to the Pleasure Principle: Enjoying yourself pays off twice. You get the immediate pleasure, and you also get better health.

Q. So doing things that are good for us feels good.

A. It's built into our nature. If evolution wanted to ensure certain behaviors, it could make either the absence of them very painful or the presence of them very pleasurable. We evolved with pleasure centers in our brain to reward us for doing things that fostered survival. For example, our sweet tooth evolved to guide our ancestors toward ripe fruits, which are ready sources of energy and certain vitamins. Our taste for fatty foods, rich in calories, helped ensure our survival during times of famine. Nowadays, while there are exceptions, enjoying food, sex, sleep, friends, work and family is our innate guide to health.

At the same time, I acknowledge that there are unhealthy pleasures. No matter how much you love to smoke, there's ample evidence that it's not healthy for you. No matter how much you savor the taste of Scotch, drinking a quart a day is bad. The fortunate thing is that *most* of the natural pleasures that we evolved to seek out have added benefits in that they also seem to promote our health.

Q. How is the Pleasure Principle different from mere hedonism, the impulse to do it if it feels good?

A. It isn't all simple selfish pleasures. We found that some of the most enriching things in people's lives are selfless pleasures. Whether it's caring for pets, ecology, loved ones, or the homeless, the things that take people beyond themselves are often intensely satisfying and, at the same time, have measurable health benefits.

On the other hand, there's nothing wrong with cultivating sensual and mental enjoyments. Our culture seems to be filled with overindulgence, yet many people don't get their minimum daily requirement of natural sensory pleasures. It's possible for people to get up and shuffle off to work barely noticing the nature around them. To spend all day indoors and never see the sun rise or set. To seldom be touched. To wolf down food and hardly taste or enjoy it.

To not listen to natural sounds or pleasant music. This deprivation is at a cost to one's well-being.

Q. Are there any concrete rewards that come from taking time to smell the roses?

A. Research has shown that ordinary pleasures can have dramatic effects on health. A German study found that a group of students who took time out for daily saunas had less than half as many colds over six months as a group that did not. Another study showed that patients recovering from gallbladder surgery spent an average of one day less in the hospital, had fewer complications and asked for less pain medication if they were given a room that looked out on trees rather than a brick wall.

When investigators piped Brahms into an operating room during surgery, patients needed only half the sedative. Gazing at fish in an aquarium lowered the blood pressure of patients with hypertension. Taking a daily siesta may decrease the risk of heart attack by as much as a third. Being touched can stabilize heart rate—even, at times, for patients who are in a coma. Smelling pleasant scents may improve moods. Getting outside and enjoying the bright natural lighting may help relieve depression. These are all clues that we evolved to seek out natural sensual pleasures.

Q. But the workaday world isn't set up for noontime siestas and soft violins. What practical advice do you have for guys in the business arena?

A. It doesn't take a tremendous amount of time to enrich your life with healthy pleasures. Maybe it's just taking brisk walks outside and really involving yourself in that and enjoying it. It takes only a little more time to really savor your food or notice the smells or aromas around you. If somebody was to say, "I'm going to skip my lunch today and go out and see a funny movie," a lot of people would frown and think he's really goofing off. And yet laughing can raise levels of antibodies that help defend us against colds and respiratory tract infections.

Q. In a balanced life, where do healthy habits, such as regular exercise and eating well, fit in?

A. The latest fitness research suggests that the greatest gains come from modest amounts of daily exercise. I think a balanced view is that health is a tool. That is, it's something we maintain in order to help us achieve something else in our lives.

Q. Do you practice what you preach?

A. Well, I used to play with my son and think about all the work I should be doing instead. Now I understand that playing with him is one of the most productive things that I can possibly do. So the answer is, yes, I'm trying to incorporate this into my life. One of the principles of healthy pleasures is that none of us is perfect. I don't have to lay that on myself. So I take very small steps. These daily enjoyments not only are the things that enrich my life but also actually are some of the best ways to stay healthy.

—John Volmer

15 Roads to Rapid Relaxation

Relax your body. Relax your mind. Here's how—from deep breathing to sports to sex.

We once read an article on ways to unwind that recommended sticking a strip of cellophane tape across your brow so you could monitor your frowns. Right. You'd be the calmest clown at the office. Then there was the book that suggested destressing by taking a siesta after lunch. Which makes us wonder: Have these stress experts ever held an actual job?

In the real world, dealing with pressures at work and at home requires an arsenal of *practical* stress solutions. Here are 15.

1. Blow it off. Deep, slow breathing can often calm the fight-or-flight response during periods of big-time stress. Usually, it takes only a few seconds to feel the difference. Simply breathe in through your nose while comfortably expanding first your abdomen and then your rib cage. (Imagine that you're inflating a beach ball inside your gut, through your navel.) Then release the breath through your nose (more slowly than you let it in) and silently say, "Relax."

2. Quick, release. In three minutes' time, you can do this to relax your muscles: (1) Sit and close your eyes; (2) inhale, and hold that breath for about 6 seconds while tensing as many muscles as you can; (3) exhale with a whoosh and let your body go limp, then breathe rhythmically for about 20 seconds; (4) repeat twice, and after the third release, relax for a minute, concentrating on a peaceful thought.

3. Make love, not warily. Sex is a good stress reliever. Most people experience a fairly profound relaxation following lovemaking. And since good sex can strengthen a relationship and boost your self-esteem, it's one of the healthiest ways to unwind.

4. Crack up before you crack. A good laugh may break up even teeth-clenching tension. Research indicates that laughter prompts the brain to release endorphins, the body's natural pain relievers. One trick you can use is to keep a tape of your favorite comedian in the glove compartment as an emergency kit for the day when you're late for work, the air conditioner is broken, and the freeway has turned into a parking lot. It works.

5. Get into hot water. "Hot baths are the oldest form of tranquilizer known," says Richard Gubner, M.D., medical director of Safety Harbor Spa and Fitness Center in Florida. He recommends soaking in water that's about 100° to 102°F—in other words, a little warmer than you are—for no more than 15 minutes. A warm shower can help, too.

6. Try some Jacu-pressure. If you have access to a Jacuzzi, try this: Instead of letting the water jets hit you in the back, slide down a bit so they pummel your neck and upper shoulders. In combination with the warm water, this gentle massage works miracles. If you can manage it without drowning yourself, let the jets on the other side soothe the soles of your feet.

7. Chill your head, not a cocktail. Instead of an after-work cocktail, try a glass of water or juice followed by ten minutes of quiet time, preferably in a quiet place with your eyes closed. Explain to those you live with that you need this little reentry period before dealing with leaky toilets, overdue bills and the fact that Junior broke Mrs. DePietro's kitchen window with a baseball.

8. Walk it off. When possible, don't schedule business lunches. Use lunch as a psychological break, a time to balance out the morning and afternoon. Eat by yourself, and try to concentrate on eating slowly. A noon nap is probably out of the question, but you should be able to take a little walk. People in a study at California State University said a brisk 10-minute walk made them feel less tense for up to two hours. "Less tense" in this case didn't mean sedated; they said they felt energized by the walks. Another study found that a 15-minute walk can have a greater calming effect than a tranquilizer.

9. Talk to yourself. It's not a sign you're crazy. In fact, it could help you avoid ending up that way. A private dialogue with your ego is a helpful way to handle stress. "You are less likely to have tunnel vision about a problem when you give yourself a chance to hear, and question and think out what you're saying to yourself," says New York psychologist Richard Sackett, Ph.D. In a survey of 208 adults, talking with oneself ranked among the top ten forms of consolation.

10. Don't "awfulize." If you hear yourself saying something like "What a colossal disaster!" on a regular basis, you're probably "awfulizing." If you have to, picture yourself living in Bangladesh during the flood season in order to understand that your kid spilling grape juice on the car seat is *not* a catastrophe.

11. Turn on the tunes and kick back. Some experts say that music for relaxation should be slow, quiet and instrumental. But don't despair if you get bored with Brahms or feel like punching someone after listening to drippy New Age music. Cheryl Maranto, Ph.D., president of the National Association for Music Therapy, says the two most important characteristics of tranquilizing music are "familiarity and preference." That means Motown or Mingus, Ella or *Exile on Main Street*—whatever makes you happy.

12. Use the gym as a dandy rescue. Regular exercise is probably the single most practical way to throw off tension. Exercising for 40 minutes can reduce stress for up to three hours afterward, whereas an equal period of rest and relaxation lowers stress for only 20 minutes, according to John Ragland, Ph.D., of the sports psychology laboratory at the University of Wisconsin. The more stressed you are, the more mellow you'll feel after exercise.

13. Take time to do nothing. It's hard to go from trying to do three things at once to doing nothing at all. But everyone needs some white space on their calendar. "Downtime can be very uplifting," notes Cliff Mangan, Ph.D., a Temple University psychologist. "If you don't have time for yourself and yourself alone, you'll be tense, irritable and anxious, which is bound to affect others. So in that respect, it's not selfish to be selfish."

14. Give the world permission to be imperfect. "Perfectionism is the world's greatest con game," writes David Burns, M.D., in his book *Feeling Good*. "It promises riches and delivers misery." In a study of more than 700 people, Dr. Burns discovered that perfectionists perfect only distress and dissatisfaction with their careers and personal lives. For all their striving, he found no evidence that they were more successful than their peers. "It's important to recognize that 100 percent is unattainable," advises University of Wisconsin psychologist Asher Pacht, Ph.D. "Settle for 90 percent and recognize that it's a pretty damned good accomplishment."

That's the spirit of compromise you need to keep in mind when tackling stress. But even if you follow every one of these tips and tricks, you'll probably feel wired every once in a while. It's just a natural fact, Jack. The human animal evolved to operate at peak efficiency under a certain degree of stress. Without stress, we'd probably all be asleep at our desk by 2:00 P.M. The idea is simply to balance the excess stress with some deliberate mellowness.

15. Call in a pro. If you can't control stress naturally, don't suffer in silence. Talk to your doctor. There are several new drugs that can help control anxiety without turning you into a zombie.

—Michael Busey

Take a Break—To Bake

Saunas offer a hot way to relax. Here are the basics of Scandinavia's favorite pastime.

The first time I took a sauna was with two neighborhood buddies in the back of a 1964 Pontiac four-door sedan. It was a sweltering mid-July afternoon, and boredom was driving us to creative entertainments.

The challenge: We were to sit inside, windows tight, until someone cried uncle. Heat rose in waves from the macadam driveway as we piled in for self-torture. Sweat beaded on our skin and quickly formed rivers that pooled in the depressions of the vinyl seat. What I remember isn't how long we suffered or who finally gave in, but how unprepared we were for the shock that followed.

We planned to blast out of the car and dive into the Eckerts' pool for a bracing cool-off. But the real surprise came when we opened the door and found that a 90-degree day could feel like ice. We're talking gooseflesh and uncontrolled shivers in the midafternoon sun. The pool felt soothing by comparison. It took several minutes for our internal thermometers to register the pool water cold and the air temperature warm. What a strange sensation!

Who knows, maybe the sauna was invented by such idle creativity; its origin is shrouded in mystery and lore. The Finns argue that they were the first to sauna, although they can't pinpoint the date more accurately than one, maybe two, millennia ago. The Swedes, Norwegians and Danes make similar claims. In any case, the sauna is as much a part of life in Scandinavia as "Monday Night Football" is in America. Rural settlers in frozen Norse countries would construct a sauna before tackling less important structures—like houses and barns. For these folks, the sauna is a place where life's worries evaporate like the *loyly*—a Finnish word that means both "steam which rises from the stones" and "soul."

Since my chance exposure to the experience in the Eckerts' driveway, I, too, have become a devotee. I believe that a winter holiday isn't complete without at least one session. It's a wonderfully hedonistic way to relax in the company of friends or family. There are a few things you need to know to get the most out of your experience.

Heat Treat

Saunas differ from other hot baths by being nearly void of moisture, which means a person can bake at higher temperatures comfortably. Ideal heat runs from 190° to 200°F, although temperatures as high as 280° are possible. (The boiling point of water, remember, is a cool 212° by comparison.) Most hot tubs hover at a lukewarm 100°, while steam baths rarely top 120°.

Although purists may swear that a wood-fired sauna is the only true kind, the saunas you'll encounter at resort areas, both here and abroad, are usually heated by electricity. Purism aside, the principle is the same as that for wood-heated saunas: Radiant heat from the main heat source warms not the room but a pile of stones atop the heater. The stones, in turn, make the sauna hot by convection. Convection heat is gentler and more consistent than the furnacelike blast of radiant heat.

The best time for a sauna is after an active day outdoors and before the evening meal. If you insist on a sauna after eating, wait at least an hour: After a meal, blood first shunts to the digestive tract, and if sauna heat is enticing the remaining blood to your skin's surface, it may cause a dangerous oxygen deficiency to vital organs, such as the heart and brain. Presauna cocktails are not a good idea, since alcohol-induced drowsiness could put you to sleep (and if nobody finds you snoozing there, it could be a *very* long sleep).

My favorite après-ski schedule is sauna at 5:00 P.M., a cocktail at around 6:30, and dinner at 7:30 or 8:00. That gives me enough time to rest, sauna and catch a second wind before the evening gets rolling.

It's important to warm the sauna and let it "ripen" before entering. That means turning on the heater when you return from skiing, or scheduling a sauna time so your host can fire it up for you. Most saunas have a one-hour timer switch. Turn it to the maximum setting and you'll have plenty of time to change and relax while it's toasting.

175 Degrees

The sauna is ripe when the mercury rises to at least 175°F and the humidity drops below 10 percent. High-tech saunas have a thermometer and a hygrometer mounted inside so you can tell when things are just so. In any case, an hour of preheating virtually guarantees a suitable atmosphere.

It's a good idea to drink a glass of water to stave off dehydration before heading in. Since the name of the game is profuse sweating through gaping pores, it's best to remove all sunscreen, makeup and moisturizing creams or oils, all of which tend to cake on your skin and clog pores.

About clothing: Don't wear any, if possible, but you'd better check out the local customs before bursting in buck naked. (Some resorts avoid any indelicacies by having separate saunas for men and women.) Wearing a loose towel is the next best thing to bathing naked, with swimsuits a distant third.

WHAT THE DOCTOR ORDERED?

The greatest quality of the sauna, of course, is that it makes you feel so damn good, so loose, so relaxed. It's as if you've cooked the tension right out. While most agree on these feel-good qualities, it's harder to support some of the more tangible health claims that aficionados make. Let's consider a few.

Weight loss. You'll melt off some weight from all the sweating you do in a sauna, but the consensus is that any change you may notice in the scale afterward should be credited to dehydration—not fat loss.

Cleaning toxins from the body. The theory is that a sauna increases the loss of nitrogen through the skin and speeds up the elimination of waste usually removed by the kidneys and excreted in the urine. That sounds good, but dermatologists say there's no clinical evidence proving that sweating eliminates significant amounts of toxic wastes from the skin.

Improving the complexion. It just ain't so, unfortunately. Heat *irritates* conditions like acne and urticaria, according to skin doctors. There are dermatologists who'll prescribe sauna baths for skin problems related to stress, but that's about as far as it goes.

Leave certain items behind. Watches and rings not only thwart the bareness ideal, they also can sear your skin. Ditto for eyeglasses: Metal frames burn, plastic ones deform. Take out your contacts, because the low humidity can dry them and irritate your eyes.

What you should take to the dressing room is a towel or two, soap, shampoo, shower shoes, a dressing robe and maybe a bath brush (the modern equivalent of a birch whisk). If there's no bucket and ladle in the sauna, take a plastic cup of water inside for sprinkling the rocks to make steam.

Those are the basics. Now that you're ready for your heat treat, here's a step-by-step guide to the fine points of sauna pleasure.

1. Sit or lie on the lowest bench until you get used to the heat (usually about five minutes). Then move up, if you like, to one of the higher benches. Since heat rises, a prone position will provide more even heating than sitting. Relax. Unwind. Avoid unnecessary movements and conversation. Your body will be bathed in a layer of perspiration in a matter of moments.

2. Once you're sweating, sprinkle a little water onto the rock pile. You'll sense an increase in heat and a tingling sensation on your skin. The temperature actually stays constant, but you feel hotter because there's more humidity. The added moisture inhibits sweat evaporation and stimulates your pores to contract momentarily—thus the quivering skin. Don't overdo it with the sprinkles. The idea is to stimulate the skin with humidity, then let the air become dry once again. Too much water spoils the sauna environment and drives bathers out prematurely.

3. For the full treatment, you'll want to try whisking. Truly. So maybe it sounds like some masochistic perversion, but don't knock it until you've tried it. Traditionally, the bather beats his skin with a whisk made from light, leafy birch branches. This stimulates surface capillaries to dilate and heightens the tingling effect begun by the steam treatment. You can get the same effects by rubbing your skin briskly with a rough towel or soft bath brush.

4. Next, step outside and into a warm shower to wash off the dirt and dead skin loosened by perspiring and whisking. Rinse with warm water, rest in the cooler air for a few minutes then skip to Step 6—or return to the sauna and try Step 5 for the maddest act in sauna lore.

5. Take the plunge. Once you've warmed up again, treat yourself to one of the wildest sensory experiences you can have without breaking the law—the ice plunge. There are several variations: jumping into waist-deep water through a hole cut in lake ice, rolling in a snowbank, hopping into a plunge tank or taking a cold shower. The secret is commitment. You can't hesitate once you've left the sauna or your skin will chill slowly and you'll miss the treat. When your skin makes contact with the cold water (or snow), your pores *slam* shut, creating a total body wave sensation.

Don't lollygag in the cold. Either move quickly to Step 6 or hop back in the sauna, warm up and try the plunge as many times as you like. One caution: If you're bathing in a public facility such as a hotel and plan a naked roll in the snow, make sure the outside door doesn't close and lock behind you. Nothing ruins total relaxation like a naked dash through a crowded lobby.

6. Although it feels relaxing, your body reads a sauna session as a bout of heavy exercise—sweating, elevated heartbeat, systemic surprises—so you should rest afterward. The best dressing rooms have a place to recline on lounges and read the paper, nap or just zone out. While your pores recover from all that dilating and contracting, let the air dry your skin for 20 to 30 minutes to be sure you've stopped sweating before dressing.

Ideally, you shouldn't take a sauna when pressed for time, but if the need for a quickie should arise, perspiration, washing and recovery provide the most significant physical benefits. The other steps are mostly for fun.

On a cautionary note, don't take a sauna when suffering an illness, because it adds systemic stress. So forget about "sweating out" that cold or flu. And further, certain people need to approach saunas slowly and cautiously, perhaps with a physician's approval. Folks over age 60 are in a high-risk group for undiagnosed heart disease. The sauna's no place to find out. Children may prefer using the lower benches for a shorter amount of time, because their smaller mass-to-surface-area ratio makes them overheat faster than adults.

Enjoy yourself for however long it feels comfortable. Leave immediately if you feel faint or sense an irregular heartbeat. If that happens, sit in the dressing room and sip water until you recover. Don't try to outlast your pals: Relax, don't compete.

—*Don Cuerdon*

Swooosh...Thwack

The aim of archery is to coordinate body and mind. This chapter targets the details of getting started.

Standing in the Olympic Stadium in Seoul, Jay Barrs could hear his heart thumping above the cheering and applause. One more bull's-eye to win a gold medal, he told himself, drawing back his bow to full tension with a steady grip.

Looking through the sight, his eyes were focused on the target, but he wasn't really seeing it. Effortlessly, he released the arrow and watched as it caught the center spot for the gold.

Archery is a complex and intriguing sport, as much mental as physical. "Being able to hit the target consistently requires focus—the ability to shut out a good deal of conscious thought," says Tim Strickland, an Olympic archery trainer.

Aim with the Brain

In sports, this focus is known as "the zone"—an elevated state of psycho-athletic awareness where your body and mind perform their best without any conscious effort. "When you're in the zone, you're still in this reality, but you're capable of watching yourself perform without any evaluation," says Keith Henschen, P.Ed., director of the applied sports psychology program at the University of Utah. He says zone performance is governed by the right hemisphere of an athlete's brain, and it comes into play when the normally dominant analytical left hemisphere cedes control.

You don't have to be a world-class competitor to hit the zone. Anyone can do it, and archery is one of the best ways to learn. But first you have to master the basics of stance (straddle the shooting line with your feet shoulder-width apart, your back foot parallel to the line, and your forward foot at a 45-degree angle to it); of anchoring the arrow, at full draw, to a fixed point on your face (and keeping your thumb under your jaw so the string hits your chin and the tip of your nose); and of sighting the target (you never take your eyes off the bull's-eye, and you hold a follow-through position until the arrow hits).

Where to Get Started

If you want to take up archery, the way to start is to join a local group. There are clubs in many cities and towns in America; most are members of the National Archery Association (NAA), the country's official amateur archery organization. To locate the club nearest you, contact the NAA at 1750 East Boulder Street, Colorado Springs, CO 80909.

Equipment doesn't require a big investment. You can get fully outfitted for $300 to $800, including bow, arrows and sight. Beyond that, all you need is finger protectors and an arm guard.

Should you find you can hit the bull's-eye with some regularity, you may want to try your hand at competition. There are local tournaments at all skill levels, usually Standard 600 or Standard 900 rounds, where archers launch 60 or 90 shafts from four different distances. Get really good and you can try for the Outdoor Nationals (held every August in Oxford, Ohio), which shoot the same rounds as the Olympic Games.

But the great thing about archery is that you don't have to compete to discover the deep satisfaction of the sport. When it comes to hitting the zone, you have no one to beat but yourself.

—*John F. Hernandez*

The Basics of Booze

Can alcohol be part of a normal, healthy life? Yes, provided you follow these rules.

Everyone knows what wise pundits barkeeps are. So needless to say, we sat up and blinked when the American Bartenders' Association offered this prediction for the 1990s: "Healthy food, moderation and quality will be deciding factors on where, when and how consumers choose to indulge and celebrate."

Actually, we worry a little that the part about healthy food will mean the demise of the Beer-Nuts and pickled eggs at our favorite tavern, but moderation and quality sound pretty smart to us. If you're going to drink, you might as well drink the good stuff, but whether you quaff Coors or Courvoisier, moderation is a secret of successful imbibing. Another is to know what you're getting into before you let the genie out of the bottle.

Here are some of the best tips we know for healthy drinking. Consider them something along the lines of a package insert for using what's fermented or distilled.

Have a slow hand. Many men end up drunk for the simple reason that they didn't give their first drink enough time to kick in before ordering up a second or third. It takes 20 to 30 minutes for alcohol to do its thing, so wait *at least* that long before having another.

Rotate your days of wine and roses. You really shouldn't drink seven days a week, even if you only have a beer or two. Daily drinkers can unknowingly build up a tolerance to alcohol and may gradually increase intake to realize the feelings they used to experience on smaller doses.

After the buzz, cut. The amount you can drink in an hour without getting smashed varies according to body weight, mood, what you've eaten and other factors. To make it simple, limiting yourself to one drink an hour, the rate at which most people metabolize alcohol, will help prevent you from becoming intoxicated. As researchers note, a "drink" is the equivalent of ½ ounce of pure alcohol, the amount contained in one 12-ounce can of beer, a 1-ounce shot of 80-proof liquor or a 4-ounce glass of most wines.

Count to two. Many alcoholism experts, including Arthur Klatsky, M.D., chief of cardiology at Kaiser Permanente Medical Center in Oakland, California, define moderate drinking as two or fewer drinks daily. Some research shows that at three drinks a day, the risk for alcohol-related problems—in particular, higher blood pressure and higher mortality rates—starts to rise.

Avoid the grape escape. Alcohol is not an antidepressant. If you've got the blues, booze will "provide only momentary relief that keeps you from tackling your problems," says Ethan Gorenstein, Ph.D., assistant professor of clinical psychology at Columbia University. Using alcohol as a cure is the first step toward making drinking a disease.

Don't drink to destress. Rather than relieving stress, drinking can actually increase anxiety. If you're going through a particularly tough time, you should be having two drinks *fewer* per week. Judith Wurtman, Ph.D., a researcher at MIT, recommends drinking little or no alcohol on a day when you know you're going to face a stressful situation.

Stay out of New Hampshire. Those folks up there are a bad influence. Their annual beer consumption—51 gallons per person—is the highest in the United States.

Read tomorrow's weather forecast. The hotter it gets and more active you are under the sun, the more trouble alcohol can cause. Booze fast-forwards dehydration, says Danny Wheat, an assistant trainer for the Texas Rangers. His team often plays in 100°-plus conditions in Arlington, Texas. "We stress to players that the night before a day game, they should limit alcohol consumption," he says.

Don't guzzle beer to quench a thirst. You've just worked out or finished a ballgame. You've got a powerful thirst, and those kegs are glistening in the sun. Wait. Do one thing at a time. Drink water to replace your sweat loss first. Beer is a lousy thirst-quencher in part because it inhibits the release of a hormone responsible for water retention. The result: frequent urination, leading to fluid *loss* rather than fluid replacement, explains nutritionist and registered dietitian Nancy Clark. Not to mention the fact that you may inadvertently end up loaded and bloated on a few hundred unnecessary calories.

Drink from a glass. Pour your beer into a glass or mug to let some of the carbonation disperse. You won't get that bloated feeling as quickly as you would have if you'd drunk from the bottle.

Train your waiter. Order beer by the glass, not the pitcher; you'll probably drink less.

Slow down the stein way. Those hinged lids on German beer steins aren't just for show. They keep the beer fresh for leisurely drinking.

Do not challenge John Goodman to a drinking contest. With few exceptions, there's no way a 150-pounder can go one-on-one with a 250-pound drinker and wake up the winner. So scale down your drinks. To come out even, the 150-pounder can handle about half the alcohol of the 250-pounder.

Play the percentages. No-alcohol beers actually have a small percentage of alcohol, under 0.5 percent by law, compared with 4 percent content for regular beer and 3 percent for light. If you want a beer that truly contains no alcohol, look for one labeled "alcohol-free."

Be a jigger bug. Unless you're a bartender who can rely entirely upon eye when measuring hard liquor into a drink, use a shot glass or jigger. If you pour straight from bottle to glass, you'll probably put in too much.

Have a cool one, not a cold one. The Europeans trash us for drinking beer cold. There may be more than snobbery involved. The closer to room temperature beer is, the better you can smell the malt, hops and yeast as you hoist it. Chilling, on the other hand, takes your nose out of play and may lead to guzzling. Buy a good brand of beer and enjoy it on the room-temperature side of cold. About 45° to 50° is ideal for most brands.

Order ice. A martini on the rocks is less potent than one served straight up, where there's no ice to melt and water down the drink. A frozen margarita is less potent than one served on the rocks: There's more water in all the crushed ice.

Party smartly. At a party, follow each drink with a glass of mineral water or soda. You'll always have something in your hand to sip, but you'll be getting half the liquor and calories you otherwise would. No-calorie carbonated mineral water and lime looks just like a 170-calorie gin and tonic. You'll also counteract alcohol's dehydrating actions.

Eat, then drink. Drinking only on a full stomach is "probably the single best thing you can do, besides drinking less, to reduce the severity of a hangover," says Mack Mitchell, M.D., vice-president of the Alcoholic Beverage Medical Research Foundation. "Food slows the absorption of alcohol, and the slower you absorb it, the less alcohol actually reaches the brain." The kind of food you eat doesn't matter much.

Scream not for ice cream. Latest drink to avoid: The hummer— rum, Kahlúa and vodka, with Häagen-Dazs thrown into a blender. You hardly taste the alcohol when you blend it with ice cream. Also, you'll get fat while you're getting drunk: A pint of Häagen-Dazs used this way makes only three or four drinks. If you start seeing pink elephants, it may be your own expanding trunk.

Clear the air. Avoid smoky bars. A substance called acetaldehyde is found in alcohol *and* tobacco smoke, and it can make a bad hangover worse. There are now bars for folks who like to drink smoke-free. One in New York is called Nosmo King.

Pass on the gas. Drinking bubbly beverages when you're drinking alcohol increases the rate at which alcohol is absorbed. Carbonation helps spread alcohol through the wall of your digestive tract, putting it into your bloodstream more quickly. Water or citrus juice is a better mixer than soda, again, particularly for preventing hangovers.

Bag the doggie. That image of a St. Bernard carrying brandy down the slopes to a half-frozen skier is medically slippery: Alcohol increases blood flow to the skin, giving you the immediate perception of warmth. But that heat is soon lost to the air, reducing your core body temperature. In short, alcohol makes you colder.

Say no to a nightcap. Alcohol makes for a poor sleeping potion because it disrupts sleep patterns. You may doze off initially, but in a few hours the effects will wear off and your body will slide into withdrawal, waking you up. If you have insomnia, avoid drinking at dinner and throughout the rest of the evening, suggests Michael Stevenson, Ph.D., a psychologist and sleep disorders specialist in Mission Hills, California. Men who snore should also skip nightcaps: "Alcohol before bed makes snoring worse," says Earl V. Dunn, M.D., a Toronto sleep specialist.

Wine down the calories. "I have found I really appreciate a good glass of wine after a couple of days of abstention," James Suckling, senior editor of *The Wine Spectator*, has noticed. He's a fan of low-alcohol wines and has suggested switching from a full-bodied chardonnay (14 percent alcohol) to a traditional German Kabinett or Spatlese (10 percent or lower).

Watch your blood pressure. If you have high blood pressure, take it easy on the alcohol. A liquor cabinet full of studies has shown that heavier drinkers show greater increases in blood pressure and moderate drinkers show smaller increases. "Two drinks or fewer a day will probably have no detrimental effect on blood pressure, but when you go beyond that, you're looking for trouble," says Norman Kaplan, M.D., of the University of Texas Health Science Center at Dallas

Southwestern Medical School. A heavy drinker with high blood pressure who stops altogether may see his pressure drop 10 to 25 points.

Protect your tummy. Heartburn or ulcer problems may flare up after you drink wine and beer. They make the stomach secrete more acids, further irritating the inner lining.

Prevent a bout with gout. If you suffer from gout, avoid alcohol, says Gary Stoehr, a University of Pittsburgh pharmacist. Alcohol seems to increase uric acid production, which can lead to gout attacks. Beer may be particularly undesirable because it is higher in a food substance called purine than wine or other spirits. If you drink, minimize your risk of a reaction by following this tip from Felix O. Kolb, M.D., of the University of California–San Francisco School of Medicine: "Drink slowly and buffer wine with readily absorbed carbohydrates such as crackers, fruit and cheeses."

Try half-and-half. Order your cocktails with the alcohol on the side so you can mix your drink at your own pace. Pour half the shot into your mixer, and when that's gone, order another glass of mixer and add the rest of the alcohol.

Stay dry when you fly. Drinking on a flight ups your chances of suffering jet lag. "The cabin atmosphere contributes to dehydration," says Timothy Monk, Ph.D., a jet lag specialist at the University of Pittsburgh. "Alcohol is a diuretic and will make you even drier. The best thing to do is drink fruit juice or decaffeinated soda."

Reason #4,763 not to drink and drive. A study by two Mississippi State University psychologists suggests moderate drinkers are even more likely than intoxicated ones to feel bold and self-assured about passing in the fast lane and driving at high speeds. Most people suffer some impairment of driving skills after only two drinks.

—*Glenn Deutsch*

PART 4

Man-to-Man Talk

Men Learn the Darndest Things

There are certain rules men live by—as silly as they sometimes are. Why, for instance, can't guys ever stop to ask directions?

When the movie *E.T.* first came out, a woman I know was surprised that her husband had shed a tear or two during the scene where the alien munchkin dies. This same guy, see, hadn't so much as misted an eye at *Terms of Endearment,* but a kid's movie got him where he lived.

That's not so odd, I said. Her husband was just following the rules: Guys must stay strong and tear-free through tragedies but are permitted to cry over the death of a pet (and E.T. was essentially Old Yeller from outer space). The only time I ever saw my father cry was the day we buried our dog: As we lowered Duke into a hole in the backyard, he hung his head and bawled.

Unspoken Rules

Men follow a covert propriety—a set of unspoken rules that governs our ways and defines what it is to be male. It's more than just knowing when it's okay for a red-blooded guy to cry; there are dozens of inner directives that tell us how to act like a man.

Where do these bylaws come from? From everywhere: Dad, first-grade readers, coaches, the Hardy Boys, baseball players, Ben Cartwright, older brothers, the Boy Scouts, Ozzie Nelson, and just hanging out with the guys.

Some anthropologists say the codes we follow today were set down way back when men got together to paint bison on the walls of caves. "Many of these behaviors have been selected by evolution," explains Warren Farrell, Ph.D., author of the book *Why Men Are the Way They Are.* "For example, it's a rule that men are supposed to be tough and protect women. This traces back to ancient times, when if women bred with men who were gentle and sensitive, those guys got wiped out by invading tribes. The men who were able to bash in some enemy skulls and save themselves and their women and children were the ones whose genes were passed on."

For modern men, we've compiled a brief list of those unspoken guidelines. These rules look fairly ridiculous on paper, but now that they're documented, you can show them to your wife or girlfriend and say, "See, honey, I'm not the only one who does this stuff. . . ."

• On car trips with the family, never ask for directions when you're lost. *Just keep driving aimlessly around, searching for the mysterious Lost Street of the Damned. Navigate by the seat of your pants, like the great explorers of old.*

• But it's okay to stop for directions when driving with another guy. *He won't sit patiently as you pass the same McDonald's for the third time.*

• Inch forward at stoplights to keep up with the guys in the cars on both sides. *It's all about who's out in front.*

• Even if you don't know a hubcap from a distributor cap, never admit you're a stranger to the male domain of auto mechanics. *If your car won't run and you're at a loss for words, try "Could be a cracked ring. Have you checked the compression?"*

• A real man doesn't need the instruction sheet to figure out something as simple as programming his new VCR. *But to cook something as simple as oatmeal, a guy will follow the recipe with the exactitude of a chemical engineer.*

• Don't confess that you know little, and couldn't care less, about a particular sport, especially if it's during the finals. *"Yeah, that Bo, he's really something. What a hook shot!"*

• Never admit you don't understand a political issue. *Opinions are like whiskers: You're not an adult male without them.*

• There's no need to consult *TV Guide* when there's a remote control handy. *Just dive-bomb through all 51 channels, evading commercials like flak, in the never-ending search for a suitable landing spot.*

• If you spill something on the floor, clean it up with a bath towel. *It's unmanly to get down on the floor, so just slop the towel around with your feet.*

• Never pay one of your buddies a compliment. Instead say things like "Who cuts your hair, some guy with a tomahawk?" or "Who is that awesome blonde I saw you with, and what are you going to do for a date once she meets me?" *He'll instinctively get the message that this means you value his friendship.*

• If a man cuts *you* with one of those insults, tell your wife or girl-friend that it hurt your feelings, and you'll come off more sensitive than Phil Donahue. But never reveal it to the other guy. *"Coach, when you said I was a low-life, turd-brained doofus for striking out with the bases loaded, it made me feel small and sad."*

• Never reveal anything about your true, actual, authentic, biological sex life to another guy. *Unless the guy is a urologist.*

• A man should earn as much as or more than his girlfriend or wife. He should be as tall or taller and at least as smart. Naturally, he should be able to outplay her in any activity, from Ping-Pong to chess. *Having met these requisites, he should be liberated enough to be unconcerned about such things.*

• If there are more than two urinals and one is being used, proceed to the farthest available urinal. If a line has formed, maintain proper spac-ing of at least three feet back from any guy using the urinal. *Above all, if nothing happens within 30 seconds, don't just stand there like a geek. Flush the toilet and walk away.*

• When you're in the men's room alone, you needn't wash your hands when you're done. *But if another guy is in there, you scrub your hands like a brain surgeon.*

• If you can't take it (whatever "it" might be), you're not a man. *Maybe you're scared of roller coasters, but if your buddies want to go on one, you'd better gird up your loins and groan through the zero-Gs, or you'll never hear the end of it.*

• Ignore or deny physical pain. *As comedian Billy Crystal reports, "Mike Tyson once hit Trevor Berbick so hard, Trevor did the dance Ann-Margret did in* Bye Bye, Birdie. *Did he hurt you, Trevor? 'I was stunned, that's all, stunned.' "*

• Never openly display a broken heart caused by a woman or discuss it with other guys. *That's between you, your six-pack, and your collection of Frank Sinatra records.*

• Don't tell another man your deepest hopes or fears. *That's like saying, "How do you like my suit of armor? It's only got two weak spots in it—here and here."*

• If you want to lose weight, don't even think about giving up Ben & Jerry's Chunky Monkey ice cream. *Instead, pull on those running shoes and pound those calories into submission.*

• Every guy should be hip about guns. *Hand an economics professor a Remington, and even if he's never been close to a firearm before, he'll work the action, sight down the barrel and generally act like a reincarnation of Daniel Boone.*

• If your wife or girlfriend is looking on, flip aloofly through that issue of *Playboy* as if it were a *Better Homes and Gardens* special issue on Tupperware. In a huddle of your peers, pause regularly to utter appreciative comments like "Wow! Check *that* out!" *And if you're alone, study and quantify each curve like a forensic scientist.*

• When shopping with your mate, do not trail her into the women's lingerie department. *Stand clear of those racks of silk-and-lace panties like a jet mechanic would avoid The Whirling Fan Blades of Death.*

—*Mark Canter*

What All Men Share

An anthropologist who has studied men the world over says we aren't so different after all. See what you have in common with a Masai cattleman or a New Guinea tribesman.

No matter how tough it was for you to grow up male in America (yeah, we know, you were the only Italian kid in a Polish neighborhood, or you were the smallest guy on the football team), *nothing* is worse than the hazing teenage boys in Sambia must pass through to earn their manhood, a ritual that involves shoving razor-sharp blades of saw grass up their noses.

On the other hand, boys of all cultures, from the sons of corporate headhunters to the sons of *real* headhunters, are indoctrinated with many of the same male ideals. "I've discovered there is almost a generic criterion of manhood across diverse societies," says David Gilmore, Ph.D., professor of anthropology at the State University of New York and author of *Manhood in the Making*. In his book, Gilmore explores these male role resemblances, stretching from the samurai of feudal Japan to the Samburu of east Africa, from ancient Athens to Athens, Ohio. *Men's Health* asked him to tell what it takes to be a man.

Q. What are the parallels in male images around the world?

A. Manhood is based on being competent in three things. The first is *provisioning*. A real man provides for his wife, his children and his group—whether he's a Truk fisherman or a Masai cattleman. He has to create a surplus. This is still the big one in Western society; the breadwinner, until the last couple of decades, was almost always male.

The second is *protection*. Defending your clan or country is exclusively a male duty. No nation in the world drafts women for combat. You don't send women of child-bearing age to their deaths if you want your society to go on living.

The third is *impregnating*. In many cultures, having lots of children and wives or mistresses shows that you're a real man.

Q. Why do so many cultures regard true manhood as "a prize to be won or wrested through struggle," as you say in your book?

A. Societies are fragile; they can die away and disintegrate or be taken over by their neighbors. To make the transition from boyhood to manhood, a male must display traits and skills the society needs to survive. Historically, those male roles have involved risk taking, aggressiveness, defense, strength, stoicism, competence, competitiveness and sexual proficiency. That's where the tests of manhood and the male rites of passage come in. For instance, men are not necessarily warlike—perhaps there's a little bit of the warrior in us because of the hormone testosterone—but it has to be encouraged, shaped by the culture. And cultures do this because *machismo* has helped them survive in many cases.

Q. It sounds as if you're describing a kind of natural selection—the survival of the manliest culture.

A. I wouldn't want to say that without such a model of manly behavior, a culture would surely disappear. But it certainly adds to a culture's strength under conditions of warfare, competition and environmental struggles, which have been widespread. When those threats disappear, then perhaps you don't need machismo. In fact, that's what I found: Cultures where there is no warfare, strife or economic competition don't have these same manly ideals and tests of manhood.

Q. What are some of the more unusual male rites of passage?

A. In the highlands of New Guinea, there's an area called the "semen belt" because of a number of cultures with the same peculiar ritual. I wrote about one of them, the Sambia. These people believe that a boy does not develop into a man naturally but must be masculinized by eating the semen of the adults in the tribe.

The Sambia also engage in what is probably the single most painful ritual in the world. The boys are taken into the bush and given stiff, sharp blades of saw grass, which they must shove up their nostrils until the blood gushes. The grown men greet the blood flow with a war cry, for the boys have shown disdain for their own pain and bloodshed—as they will have to do as men on the battlefield.

The Samburu of east Africa are cattle herders. The boys are put through a circumcision rite at the age of 13 or 14. Without anesthetic, their foreskins are cut off, and they are forbidden to move a muscle or cry out in pain while the circumcision is taking place. After this test, they're awarded their manhood, and then they are expected to stand up to lions and defend the tribe from attack. A real Samburu man is supposed to have at least two children and be a good cattleman and provide meat for everyone.

Q. What about in American culture?

A. Boys growing up here are directed mainly to the role of breadwinner and to the values of independence, productivity, competence and so on. But there are violent subcultures, such as inner-city gangs, where males might literally fight to the death to defend their turf.

The rites of passage for American boys are mostly symbolic. You don't actually have to defend your turf, unless you're a gang member. But guys defend their high school's honor in sports, and they take risks in all sorts of ways. Then successful men are expected to channel that drive into college, career, family and life achievements.

Q. Is there a deeper structure to these cultural resemblances? Is male behavior biological?

A. I don't believe in a universal male or female—but on the other hand, you can't discount 100 million years of evolution. Male and female sex hormones are very different, and they influence us to behave in distinct ways. Culture then takes those biological givens and exaggerates or suppresses them. Some cultures have come close to extinguishing the biological differences between men and women.

Q. We've talked about behaviors and attitudes; what about looks? Are there generic notions about "manly-looking" men?

A. Remember the Bush/Dukakis debates? Dukakis stood on a platform so he wouldn't look small next to Bush. In the United States and all around the world, it's usually tall, muscular men who are the most successful. Their size and strength goes along with the male roles of provisioning and protection. Also, women seem to be more attracted to taller men, so you can include impregnating. Feminists are outraged that men judge women first on the basis of their looks. But turn it around and ask them what they think about weak, skinny little guys. . . .

Q. What about cultures that don't fit the pattern? Are there places where manhood is of little importance to men?

A. The two that I came across are the Semai of Malaysia and the Tahitians of French Polynesia. They don't really care about the differences between men and women. There are no tests or rites of passage for the boys. They don't distinguish between a "real man" and an effeminate man—they just don't care. Men and women do pretty much the same jobs. The women are more in charge of child rearing, but both sexes cook, plant, tend animals and fish. And importantly, both these societies are not warlike.

Q. How did these two cultures cope with warfare?

A. The Semai proudly say, "We run away from danger." They don't believe in bravery. When adrenaline hits and they have the choice of fighting or fleeing, they flee.

The Tahitians long ago enclosed themselves on their bountiful island and did not engage in warfare. They avoid anger and all kinds of aggressive behavior.

Q. What was your most surprising finding?

A. The widespread emphasis on generosity, on male giving; that in most societies, men are expected to produce and give more than they take.

I think the idea that men are privileged and women are underprivileged has been overstated. The fact is, male advantage also carries with it great responsibilities and risks, one of which is to be sent off to war—50,000 men of my generation died in Vietnam. So the critique of the sex roles has to be made with a little more sensitivity to the history of their contributions to the society. I'm definitely not saying that the sacrifices of women should be belittled or ignored, only that the sacrifices of men should be acknowledged and not taken for granted.

Q. What can your research tell the average guy?

A. That it's okay to be a traditional male. That while the traditional gender roles have their limiting aspects, they have provided ways for men and women to complement each other.

Some have argued that because male and female roles are strongly influenced by culture, you can do anything you want with them—even get rid of them altogether. I don't buy that. Just because something is culturally determined doesn't mean it's dispensable. Societies have their needs. You can't just toss out male and female roles that have developed over hundreds of years; the society won't survive.

—*Russell Segal*

Fatherly Wisdom

Looking back, we realize that Dad taught us some important lessons. A survey of men reveals what these lessons are.

When I was a boy of fourteen, my father was so ignorant
I could hardly stand to have the old man around. But when
I got to be twenty-one, I was astonished at how much
he had learned in seven years.

—*Mark Twain*

Fatherly wisdom really does seem to improve with age, but of course, it's *your* age, not his, that makes the difference. Words of advice that did nothing but annoy you as a teenager can suddenly leap across the generation gap and make perfect sense when you reach your thirties. As one man, perhaps less clever but more straightforward than Twain, puts it: "At 17 I got too much of Dad's advice, especially about girls. At 37, I can't get enough."

Part of the problem all along was that Dad didn't always come right out and *say* what was on his mind. What many men remember about their father are examples of his behavior—the way he handled a particular problem or moral dilemma. In his sometimes awkward way, he knew what he was doing.

"Our fathers felt responsible for making men out of us. It was their job," says Ronald Levant, Ed.D., a psychology professor and coauthor of the book *Between Father and Child*. "Men learn life lessons and wisdom from their father, and fathers often teach those lessons by example."

Men's Health interviewed men from across the country—some friends and business acquaintances, some complete strangers—and asked them the most important lesson they learned from their father. Nearly every person interviewed had at least one story to tell; here are some of the best.

My father was giving me a lift to college, and I began griping about how I hated Spanish class so much—not to mention math—and that it made me sick just to think about it. I was about 19 or 20 at the time, and he told me something he'd never talked about before. When he was a young man, he said, working as an insurance salesman, the boss would line up all the men every morning, as if they were army recruits. He would go down the line and insult and humiliate each and every one of them. That was his way of motivating them. And that was how every day began for my father, week after week, month after month, year after year. But there was a depression on, and he was glad to have the job, he said. He'd never mentioned this before, because complaining was not in his nature. "If you get through college," he told me, "you won't have to put up with that." I got through college. And a lot of other things.

—Insurance vice-president, 51

Dad never got violent or angry; he became "disappointed" when I screwed up. He was my role model, and I wanted his approval. Boy, do I hate "disappointed."

—Advertising executive, 36

On my fourth birthday, my dad took me to Freedomland, a Wild West amusement park in the vast uncharted wilderness somewhere east of the Pecos and west of Fair Lawn, New Jersey. The last attraction of the day was a stagecoach ride, but what began as a pleasant little jaunt soon turned scary when we were bushwhacked by a band of outlaws. They chased us, hooves pounding and guns blazing. Finally, they overtook us, pulled the coach to a stop, threw open the door and held us up at gunpoint.

Naturally, I assumed they were after my Special Issue Freedomland Souvenir Tricolor Pen, so I did what any self-respecting four-year-old would have done—I cried like a banshee. It was then that my father performed the most remarkable act of bravery I'd ever seen. He looked that gang leader right in the eyes and said, "All right, fellas. That's enough."

To my astonishment, that ruthless desperado looked back at my father and mumbled, "Okay. Sorry, sir." Then he and his cutthroat gang holstered their six-shooters and hightailed it for the hills. The world was safe once again. My dad was a hero. I never forgot the feeling it gave me, and I hope I can make my own son feel that way about me someday.

—Freelance writer, 39

I remember asking him a child's question: "If I were in the street and about to get hit by a car, would you run naked out into the traffic to save me?" He said of course he would. Not just for me, but for a total stranger. I thought about this for a while. I tried to imagine my father the hero, naked and hairy, bounding across the street in the little farm town, saving lives.

—Yoga instructor, 29

The first time I wanted to dump a girlfriend, I couldn't figure out how to do it without bringing down the temple upon my head. I went to my dad and asked him, How do I break up with this girl? How do I tell her that I don't want to see her anymore? "There's no easy way," he said. And as I subsequently found out and have been continuing to find out throughout my life, he was plumb right.

—Wine merchant, 45

The only time Dad ever really *talked* to me was when I was living at home while in college and having my first heavy relationship with a girl. I was coming home late a lot, and as I stole through the front door at 4:00 one morning, Dad came out of his bedroom and took me aside. He said he was concerned about me and we should talk later. We went out to lunch the next day, but he never mentioned the previous night. It wasn't necessary for him to spout off about what was bugging him; just knowing I was keeping him up nights was enough to make me want to mend my ways.

—*Editor, 30*

My friends and I were out in the woods one day, shooting at cans with our .22 rifles. On the way out we stumbled across a wild turkey, and I impulsively shot it. Since it wasn't hunting season, we got scared and threw the carcass down a steep riverbank. When I got home, my father casually asked what I'd been doing with my gun. I didn't want to lie to him, so I blurted out the tale of the turkey. Without a word, he stood up and went into the other room to get his boots. Then he grabbed two flashlights and said, in a tone that didn't encourage further discussion, "Come on, we're going to go find it." It was cold and dark when we got back into the woods. We searched for nearly an hour, and I was just about ready to plead frostbite when I found the bird. We brought it home, dressed it and put it in the freezer.

I still love to hunt, but my father taught me a lesson I haven't forgotten. To this day, I've never killed any animal I wasn't prepared to eat.

—*Photographer, 40*

My dad told me that I should think about having more than one career in my lifetime. "Around 45 you should consider changing your career, maybe not a new field completely, but a major change that will give you new perspectives and challenges and a renewed excitement about life." Shortly after he said this, he followed his own advice and changed careers. As I approach middle age, I'm giving it a lot of thought myself.

—*Real estate salesman, 33*

My next-door adult neighbor was always picking on me. One hot summer afternoon, I was riding my new Stingray bike and cut across the edge of his finely manicured lawn. He came running out of the front door and yelled, "You little son of a bitch, you ever do that again, I'll break your f—ing neck."

My dad was just coming around the corner in the car with his window open and heard what the neighbor said. He screeched to a halt and, in a quiet but clearly angry voice, said, "Anderson, you ever talk to my kid like that again, I'm going to break *your* f—ing neck." I'd never heard my dad talk like that before, but the neighbor never bothered me again. It made me feel good to know he stood up for me.

—Press secretary, 35

He gave me this warning: "Never quit a job when you're angry." I've been tempted a few times when my ego was bruised or I felt I'd been screwed, but I've always found ways to work things out after I cooled down.

—Hospital manager, 59

My stepfather was a crackerjack car salesman, one of the best. He taught me how to avoid buying a used lemon from a private owner. "Don't talk to the seller when you're looking the car over," he told me. "Kick the tires, open the hood, get under the body, but don't say a word. Most people can't stand the silence—they get nervous and start talking, and what they often blurt out is what's *wrong* with the car. If you run your finger around the inside of the tailpipe for 30 seconds without saying anything, they'll volunteer that the car burns a little oil. It happens every time." The guy was a good psychologist in his own way, which I guess is helpful if you're a salesman. I can't tell you how many junkers I've been spared by using his routine.

—Hotel clerk, 24

He gave me some good advice about those nail-biting periods of anticipation when you're waiting to hear about a job, a lab report, an acceptance to a college. "No news isn't good news," says Dad, ever the bubble-bursting realist. "No news is . . . no news."

Obvious? Maybe. But now when I go through such anxious times, I try not to agonize, play guessing games or badger the mailman. Instead, as much as possible, I simply get on with my life. As Dad recognized, the news—good or bad—will be the same whether you worry about it or not.

—Bartender, 23

I grew up in a tightly knit community of Cuban Jews where everybody knew everybody else. We had one of everything, and so we had a village idiot, a boy no one ever got to know. One day my father took me aside for the one and only man-to-man talk we ever had, and the core of his concern turned out to be whether I was masturbating and how often. I don't remember any response on my part. But whatever I said apparently was not what he wanted to hear, because *then* he told me that masturbation was very, very dangerous and that there was no telling where it would lead, but one thing was for sure: That slow boy in our crowd was a living example of its evil ways. This was terrifying news for a boy of 12, and for a while afterward, I didn't even allow myself to *look* down there. I think this lasted a week or so.

—Commercial artist, 45

Not all lessons have the intended effect. I'll always remember the time my father spotted two teenage boys in the act of overturning a Dumpster in front of the apartment building where we lived in New York City. Punks on a lark, they were flinging discarded cartons of papers up in the air and watching the stuff float down like confetti all across the street. My father ran out and seized them by the arms and dragged them into the lobby. Then he called the police. The boys— big, leather-jacketed lugs—wept and pleaded for release. But my father was enraged and determined to carry out this moral lesson to its conclusion. I watched, terrified, from behind the marble balusters on the stairway landing as two policemen came into the lobby and calmly— even gently—escorted the boys out of there. I learned a lesson about civic responsibility that day. I also vowed never to let my father catch me if I got into trouble.

—Production manager, 38

I remember an incident when I was a kid and my father found a wallet. It had a lot of money in it. I thought, "This is great. We have all this money." But my dad called the owner and returned the wallet. I learned a sense of respect for other people's property. I never went shoplifting with my friends—walking out of a store wearing two pairs of jeans.

—College professor, 41

My father repeatedly told my three brothers and me, "Whatever you can conceive and believe, you can achieve." I heard it so often I actually believe it today.

—Carpenter, 31
—Steve Slon and Michael Lafavore

Lost in Splitsville

Divorce can be a lonely place, full of anxiety, uncertainty and self-doubt. But picking up the pieces after the lawyers leave is possible.

The man had been a prisoner of war in Vietnam. He'd suffered unspeakable fear, pain and degradation. But as awful as that experience was, the man told his psychologist, he had recently confronted something even worse: a divorce.

"In prison I could take the physical pain. I lived eight years on crutches because I broke my right leg when I bailed out. I was tortured and I found I could stand that. But the emotional test of the past few weeks has been hard to pass," the man told *Men's Health* advisor Herb Goldberg, Ph.D.

Not every man gets whacked that badly by a divorce. But nobody emerges from the experience unscathed or unchanged. Life is not one big party after your average marriage breaks up. Splitsville can be a lonely place, full of anxiety, uncertainty and self-doubt. Getting past all that takes time.

"My divorce is like a cold I can't quite shake," says Bill Miller (name changed), a Los Angeles public relations executive. "It's been two years and I feel it less nowadays, but it lingers on in my life."

Clinical psychologist Judith Wallerstein, Ph.D., who studied 60 divorced couples for her book *Second Chances,* found that ten years after divorce, half the men had serious misgivings about their decision to divorce. "Many surveys have found that it takes two or three years for both men and women to get their lives back together," she adds. Some had trouble concentrating on their work for up to two years after a split.

Rough Going

What's the message? That it's easier to stay in a lousy marriage than to face the pain of divorce? No. In fact, studies have shown that it's probably healthier in the long run to get a divorce than to stay in an insufferable relationship. Still, very few men can walk away from a bad marriage and step directly into the good life. You've got to expect that the terrain is going to be difficult, both physically and emotionally.

"Even with my training and experience as a professional counselor, I wasn't prepared for the emotional impact of divorce when it hit me," admits San Francisco psychologist Mel Krantzler, Ph.D.

Mind you, Dr. Krantzler, who went on to create a series of divorce-recovery workshops and to author *Creative Divorce,* isn't all doom and gloom: "It's up to the man what he makes of it. The consequences can be negative. They can also be very positive."

No matter what your attitude toward the proceedings, handling the day-to-day emotional baggage of divorce is hard work. Recently divorced or separated men frequently describe the way they feel in terms like "I feel suspended between the past and the future," "I'm nervous because I don't know what's in store for me in the next year" and "Despite the breakup I still feel a sense of attachment to my ex-wife."

Just about every man will go through a period of mourning following a divorce, even if he and his wife had been separated for some time. Feelings of guilt—especially if he did the leaving—and failure are normal. "Divorce is like a death in the family," says psychologist Myrna Hartley, Ph.D. "Even if you've ended up hating your wife, when the marriage ends, something important has died with it and you need to mourn its passing. It's painful to pass through this period, but you'll come out much stronger in the end."

Allow Yourself to Mourn

Skip this stage—say, by being a wildman about town—and you're inviting long-term problems like depression, warns University of Oklahoma psychologist Donald J. Bertoch, Ph.D. He recommends therapy, maintaining positive relationships with friends and family and basically refraining from making major decisions during the first post-divorce year.

The idea is to get through your grief without giving a bunch of it to your kids, family, boss, coworkers . . . and dates. "Finish the grief process before developing a new significant relationship," Dr. Bertoch says, "otherwise, it will contaminate the quality of caring and loving for the other person."

One key to successful emotional recovery is to resist the urge to blame everything that went wrong on your ex-wife. Says famed divorce lawyer Melvin Belli in his book *Divorcing*, "If I had it to do all over again here is how I would handle my own divorce: I would recognize that it takes two to make a marriage turn sour. That means that I have shared in the responsibility for my marriage ending. Not intentionally, but because I let things that were going wrong drift, and I believed everything that created arguments and tension was always the other person's fault."

Belli has had a lot of practice at this (he's been divorced four times) and he knows what he's talking about. Dr. Krantzler, who is coauthor of Belli's book, agrees. "The problem may be that *you* have been dealing with interpersonal relationships unsuccessfully. Accept that and you'll find the remedies."

Learn Your Lesson

"Divorce is an opportunity to learn the hard way how to relate to women," he adds. "It's also a place to set your priorities straight. Life's problems aren't solved by making money, owning a big house or buying new toys. The primary things are love and companionship. Divorce gives you another chance to make this discovery. If you do learn this, the rest of your life will be richer."

Along with the emotional ups and downs come physical changes. "Divorce is a major stressor, even when it's amicable, says Allan Rabinowitz, a Santa Monica stress-management expert. "If it's bitter, the impact can be that much worse. Tension soars, immunity may be weakened—possibly resulting in more colds and flus—and sleeping habits may change."

The period after a divorce may be the first time a man has lived on his own as an adult. His eating habits are almost sure to undergo a radical change, often leading to a weight loss or gain. Studies show divorced men tend to drink and smoke more, as well.

"Divorce is hard on your body," Rabinowitz concludes. "The antidote is to accept that this is a difficult time; that your symptoms are normal. And then take concrete steps, like focusing on health. Keep to an exercise program. Watch your diet in particular, because a bad one can make dealing with the stress that much harder."

The Sexual Angle

Minor sexual problems are so common after divorce that it's probably wise to expect them. A survey of 30 divorced men, published in *Sexuality Today,* showed that among men whose wives initiated the split—and in most cases it's the wife who does—impotence or premature ejaculation was common. During the first sexual encounter after the divorce, *all* the men had erectile problems, usually because they felt they were being judged by their new sex partner. The men who had initiated their divorces had fewer troubles.

"Many divorced men experience problems around dating and sex," says Bernie Zilbergeld, Ph.D., author of the book *Male Sexuality.* "A big reason is that as a marriage falls apart, so does the sex. His wife may have told him he's not a good lover, that she never had an orgasm, that he was too rough . . . too fast. He hears that he's basically an awkward sex partner and he may carry this self-image with him into dating."

Here, too, there's a cure of sorts. "If you're not functioning sexually," Dr. Zilbergeld says, "that's a clue that you haven't emotionally finished with your ex-wife. This doesn't mean you have to talk it out with her. Usually you don't." Instead, he says, step back a few paces in the mourning process and get control over those postmarital feelings. Do it on your own, with friends or with a counselor. "Once you finish with her, you can get on with developing a new, effective self-image," Dr. Zilbergeld says.

A final postdivorce problem is limited to men with children, but for them it may be the toughest hurdle of all. In about 90 percent of divorces, the mother gets custody of the kids. "If you have children," says psychologist Diane Medved, Ph.D., author of *The Case against Divorce,* "a divorce will affect you emotionally for the rest of your life."

Rich Fowler (name changed), a Phoenix engineer, agrees: "I've been divorced 12 years and, whenever I see my daughter—she's 16 now—I remember the pain I went through." Carl Vaughan (name changed), a Washington, D.C., government employee, tells a similar story: "What I most regret about my divorce—really *all* that I regret—is that it cut me off from my son. He's 15. I haven't really known him since he was 5, and that hurts."

Fashion a New Fatherhood

Here, remedies are thornier. No matter how many bad feelings the divorce stirred up, staying on at least cordial terms with your ex-wife will help make the transition easier on the children. And it's usually not a good idea to be a "Disneyland Dad," unless that's the way you were before the divorce; kids usually just want to relate to their father the way they always did. Beyond that, the best advice for divorced fathers is probably just hang loose and take each new situation as it comes. "If you're creative," Hartley says, "you'll find new relationships with your children."

Don't expect that new relationship to be inexpensive, however. Divorce can make the logistics of fathering extremely complicated. Take the case of Walt Dietrich (name changed), a Philadelphia-area executive whose 12-year-old daughter lives with him during the summer but with her mother in Minneapolis during the school year. Dietrich's effort to be a long-distance father from September through June involves numerous plane tickets, phone calls at 10:00 every weekday evening, faxing copies of report cards and the like . . . you get the picture. "It's worked well for the last three years," Dietrich says, although he realizes that soon he's going to be competing for her time at night and on weekends. "She's going to be on the phone with friends, hanging out on weekends with friends—like I did when I was a teenager," he says. "I'm already seeing a time when long distance won't be the next best thing to being there."

Given how divorce can thump a man's mind and body, not to mention those of the people around him, the rewards aren't always immediately evident. But to men who are going through a marital breakup and are having second thoughts, Dr. Rabinowitz offers some encouraging words: "You will survive. If you make the effort, you will recover. It may not be an easy process, but in the end, you'll have a more satisfying lifestyle." Divorce, he promises, "can be the key that unlocks a new, richer life."

—*Robert McGarvey*

PART 5

The Women in Our Lives

Secrets Men Keep

There are times to tell and times to clam up— do you know the difference? Sex therapist Marty Klein warns that some secrets can be damaging to a relationship.

Psssst. Can you keep a secret? Damn right you can, especially if it's one of your own. We men are notoriously stingy when it comes to revealing what's going on in our heads. We'll talk for hours about the data-retrieval speed of the new PS/2; just don't ask us to share anything really *personal*.

Keeping some things to ourselves isn't necessarily bad. We all need to defend our own little corner of private space. But Palo Alto sex therapist Marty Klein says some secrets, particularly sexual ones, can damage a relationship. "We live in a world that encourages sexual secrets," says Klein, a board member of the Society for the Scientific Study of Sex and the author of *Your Sexual Secrets: When to Keep Them, How to Share Them.* "These secrets don't always protect us or make our lives better. On the contrary, they can hold back the progress of a relationship and distort our sex lives."

Men's Health talked to Klein about when secrets should be revealed and when they're better left unspoken.

Q. When most of us think of sexual secrets, we think of things like cheating on our partner and not telling her. From your book, it's clear that your definition of *secret* is broader than that.

A. Keeping secrets is not just about lying. It's also about withholding information or arranging for people to have the wrong impression about something.

Q. Can you give an example?

A. Let's say a man has a vasectomy and he's perfectly fine about it. Four years later, he starts dating a woman who's interested in having children. She doesn't ask "Did you ever have a vasectomy?"—most people don't walk around asking that. And he doesn't mention it. So by his silence, he allows her to believe he's fertile when he isn't.

Q. I think many people would agree that's not particularly ethical. But your book makes the point that this also hurts him. How?

A. The consequences of sexual secrets are pretty wide ranging. Men who keep sexual secrets always have to fear being discovered. And if the kinds of things that they're hiding involve the way they like to be touched and the way they like to make love, then lovemaking becomes a dangerous enterprise.

This situation leads to a sense of isolation, a distance from your partner. What's really sad is that you never get to know if in fact you are loved for who you really are. There are a lot of men out there saying "Well, she *says* she loves me, but if she really knew what I was like, she wouldn't." Now it may well be that this woman would love him no matter what, but he'll never have the opportunity to find that out.

Q. Is the decision to keep secrets a conscious one?

A. I think that a lot of people don't get the personal space they need. They have to account for all of their time. They feel that they are always under somebody else's inspection. The only way they feel they can create a place where they have a time-out is by creating their own little private world.

A lot of us are not comfortable with closeness and intimacy, and we use sexual secrets to maintain that distance. If you don't want that distance, having sex secrets is going to give it to you whether you like it or not. And if you do want the distance, secrets are pretty handy.

Q. What's the most common secret men keep?

A. It's extremely common for men to masturbate. Among sex therapists, we joke that 90 percent of men masturbate and the other 10 percent are lying about it. A lot of men feel that it is either dishonorable or childish, and they hide this from their partner. What happens is that they feel guilty about it, or maybe they're afraid of getting caught, and they have to do it furtively. This is a real problem. Again, it creates distance—not the masturbating, but the hiding it.

Now I'm *not* telling every man to run and confess to his wife that he masturbates. But in many cases, if he did, it would take a lot of the pressure off.

Q. What about the role of secret fantasy?

A. Again, I don't think that everybody needs to tell all their fantasies. That could be a problem. But just acknowledging to your partner that you think about other people sexually can really be a big relief. I think that we all go around pretending that we never do this. It's obviously not true.

Q. So whether or not you open up about the problem, you have to be honest with yourself.

A. A lot of us, when we make something secret, act as if the thing has stopped existing. That's denying a part of ourselves. For example, suppose you're attracted to someone, and you decide not to tell your regular partner about it. Fine. You do that in order to make life easier for her—and for you. It's not so fine to pretend to yourself that you actually are not attracted to this person.

Q. Where does this need to sweep sexuality under the rug come from?

A. When we were young, most of us were taught that sexuality is bad. We learned that when we got our hand slapped for touching ourselves in public; we learned that when we got our mouth washed out with soap for saying "bad" words; we learned that when our parents were uncomfortable about washing us in the genital area; we learned that when we got punished for playing doctor with Suzie next door. And as a result, we learned that we have to deny our sexuality, hide it—both because we don't want to get punished and because we do want the approval.

Q. Why is there such a cloud of danger around sexuality?

A. The American culture has a conspiracy against sexuality. This is a culture that is suspicious of pleasure. We believe that the human body is fundamentally a dirty object, and that sexual energy is dangerous unless it's channeled in very particular ways. We have more rules about what's right and wrong about sex than we do about almost anything else.

Q. You say in your book that many men have things that they would like their partner to do in bed that they're afraid to ask for. Can you give an example?

A. There are so many examples of things men feel uncomfortable asking their partners for. But let's take a subtle one: Say a man likes oral sex but wishes his partner would do it a little bit differently. She does it, may even be enthusiastic about it, but she doesn't stimulate him in quite the way he likes. If the man doesn't say anything, that's a sexual secret. It's a secret because the man is withholding relevant information.

Q. What's so bad about just enjoying it her way?

A. A lot of men feel that the way *they* like it isn't really okay. They believe it isn't really okay to have a preference. The big thing is normalcy. A lot of men are concerned that maybe it's not normal to want what they want in bed; they fear that perhaps what they desire is so unusual that their partner will not only reject the particular request but will also reject them. But it's important to keep in mind that if you're with someone who loves you, that person wants to please you and wants information about how to do that.

Q. The way you describe it, the fear sounds highly irrational. But aren't there some sexual requests that might send a partner running?

A. Perhaps, but it's extremely common to fear asking for even the most ordinary sexual things. It all comes from an underlying lack of confidence that what we want sexually is okay.

I know when I go to a restaurant, I don't worry "Gee, if I order squid, my wife is going to say 'Get away from me.' " What she'll probably say is "I can't believe you eat squid. I would never eat that. But go ahead and eat it if you want."

We don't, as a rule, worry about whether we eat in a normal way. That's partly because we can see everybody eat all around us. If we could know what other people's sexual fantasies are, if we could hear the sounds people make, then we wouldn't have to keep guilty secrets about what should really be nonissues.

Q. I guess it doesn't help that our limited exposure to other people's sexuality usually comes from X-rated videos.

A. Right. We watch Wimbledon on TV, and we don't expect to be able to play tennis like Boris Becker. But when we watch X-rated videos, a lot of us expect to be able to perform that way. Besides, we forget that many of these people's "skills" are due to the magic of editing.

Q. What other common secrets are there?

A. A lot of men have performance anxiety, but they pretend that they don't. What we know about anxiety is that when you talk about it, the anxiety eases. And we also know that people are usually more anxious about things than the situation warrants.

Let's say a man has a few experiences where he doesn't get an erection in the way that he wants to. So the next time he gets into bed, typically he's afraid that he's not going to get an erection. Failing to get an erection is no big deal. But if he's really anxious about it, two things will happen. First of all, it'll be more difficult to get an erection. Second, he won't be able to deal with what's going on in a positive way. For example, if he's really wound up about how this makes him a terrible lover and how he's not a real man, he won't be able to say to his partner "Gee, that's too bad. I wonder what else we can do."

Q. That's all well and good to say. But after all, there is this woman lying there, waiting for something to happen.

A. In talking with thousands of women over the years, what comes across almost every single time is "I don't mind so much that he doesn't get it up. It's that when he doesn't get it up, he turns away from me."

Q. So in an ideal world, he'd just say . . .

A. He could say, "Look, it's not working tonight. I hope that's okay. Do you want to talk about it?" Or he might say, "I'm so stressed out. I really want to be sexual with you, but I'm not sure if I can manage an erection. I hope it'll be okay if we do something that doesn't involve intercourse." By discussing the issue, he normalizes it and also gives his partner a chance to say "It's okay."

Q. Isn't it possible that raising sensitive issues will only make things worse? How do you know if it's worth it to open up?

A. There are no guarantees. We'd all like to know that "If I do A, my partner will do B." It just doesn't work that way. And furthermore, I don't think conflict is such a bad thing. I think that if you're going to have intimacy, you're going to have conflict. The question is, is it going to be destructive or is it going to be productive?

Q. Why do we expect there to be no conflict?

A. There's a widespread belief that conflict destroys love. People have a hard time understanding that you can be angry at them and still love them. One of the things we can do is to keep reminding our partner *why* we are sharing the information: "I'm telling you this because it's driving me crazy" or "I notice that my sex drive is going down, that I've been avoiding sex with you, and I don't want to do that anymore."

Q. Give an example of a secret that's better kept a secret.

A. Sometimes an extramarital affair is better not discussed. If whatever impelled somebody to do that has been worked out and there's nothing to be gained from revealing the information, then I'd say just keep it a secret.

As another example, let's say a person has a recurring sexual fantasy about his wife's best friend. Sharing that information could be mean-spirited and destructive. Same thing with going into great detail about how she compares to his old girlfriends.

A man needs to ask himself some serious questions about his motives and goals before he reveals secrets about himself. Is it to manipulate, control or hurt his partner? Or is it honestly to get closer?

If the sharing is for negative reasons, then it's not helpful. Even under the guise of being honest, one can be hurtful. We each know where our partner is vulnerable. The key to all this is to be tender with that spot. Deep down we can tell when revealing a secret is not in the service of either a relationship goal or a personal goal—that's when you don't share.

—Steve Slon

Flash! Men and Women Are Different!

Forget everything you've learned in Politically Correct 101. There are at least 30 ways in which men and women are different.

Even those of us who are politically correct enough to skip the pink and blue baby clothes have come to admit there are differences between the sexes that can't be ignored. Reality, it turns out, is heavily laced with yin and yang. From the incidence of heart disease to the tolerance of pain to our strategies for seduction, men and women go their separate ways. Here are some facts and figures to prove it.

1. Body talk. The average adult U.S. male is 5-foot-9; the average female, 5-foot-4. He carries 1½ times as much muscle and bone as she does, and half as much fat.

2. High hopes. Men tack on an average of more than half an inch to their true height, while women subtract more than two pounds from their true weight, according to the Metropolitan Insurance Company.

3. The longevity gap. In the United States, women live 7.3 years, or 2,665 days, longer than men. At age 65, the ratio of surviving women to men is 100 to 65. Hang around. Gerontologist Steven Fox, D.O., says, "By following a healthy exercise regimen alone, men could increase their longevity by about 9 percent."

4. Yeah, but what if *Sex* magazine had done the survey? For men, money and sex are equally important, but for women, money is on their mind more often than sex, according to a survey by *Money* magazine. And more women said they *enjoy* money more than sex.

5. Tab hunters. More women than men take vitamins. An estimated 88 million women use vitamin and mineral products, compared with 81 million men.

6. The burden of proof. More than 8 percent of men are alcoholics, compared with only 3.5 percent of women, according to the National Institute on Alcohol Abuse and Alcoholism. Men can drink more than women before suffering health problems, because their metabolism of alcohol is faster.

7. "Not tonight, dear . . ." Men suffer fewer aches and pains than women, reports *USA Today*. Women feel at least one symptom of discomfort (headache, fatigue, etc.) more than 43 percent of the time, compared with men's 28 percent. Then again, men find it twice as tough to take the same amount of chronic pain as women. Being in pain is also more likely to lower a man's self-esteem than a woman's.

8. Remember the Maine vacation? Women remember better than men, and the discrepancy increases with age. In a word-recall test at Johns Hopkins Medical Institutions, men generally lagged slightly behind women; men in their late sixties scored a full 20 percent lower than did women of the same age.

9. Eye opener. Men have a weaker sense of smell than women, but are more sensitive to light.

10. Joint custody. Males in their senior year of high school are only slightly more likely to have smoked marijuana (63 percent) than are women (56 percent), according to *Drugs in American Society* by Erich Goode. However, the boys were more than twice as likely to be daily users—10 percent versus 4 percent.

11. No kidding. We all can dish it out, but who can take it? According to *Psychology Today,* men and women equally resent criticism from their mates, but men take it more to heart when their kids put them down.

12. Time's on our side. The University of Iowa asked a group of managers how they would persuade a tardy employee to show up on time. More than 60 percent of the male managers but only 37 percent of the females said they would use warnings, criticisms and ultimatums. In contrast, 30 percent of the women but only 12 percent of the men said they would try a counseling approach ("Is there anything I can do to help you get to work on time?").

13. Defense mechanism. Men are more likely than women are to favor spending money on nuclear weapons, according to *Source* magazine. Men also tend to view military defense issues in simpler terms, while women tend to have a more complex perspective.

14. Look who's talking. Men converse mostly about news events and work; women talk mostly about food and health, according to a study published in *U.S. News & World Report.*

15. Wheel difference. On average, men drive more than twice as many miles as women annually: Men average 13,412 miles; women, 6,079.

16. Can't touch this. Women are more prone than men to get ripply fat—sometimes called cellulite—on their thighs and buttocks because the fibers holding their skin to muscle are in parallel cords. This structure permits fat to bulge through and marble the skin. You seldom see cellulite on men because under the skin men have a dense mesh of fibers, which unites the fat in one smooth layer.

17. Their loss is our gain. A study of University of Michigan freshmen found that 85 percent of the women wished to lose weight; 45 percent of the men wanted to *gain* weight.

18. Sympathy for the devils. To get a date, guys tend to boast about their past accomplishments and earning potential, and to show off their cars and stereos, according to a study in the *Journal of Personality and Social Psychology*. Women more often rely on their looks and may play hard to get or display sympathy for a guy's troubles.

19. Provide and conquer. Men tend to choose a mate based on good looks. For women, a man's looks are not as important as his social status and wealth, says David Buss, Ph.D., a psychologist at the University of Michigan.

20. Close calls. Men feel nearly as much need for intimacy as women but experience it differently, according to a study done at Loyola University of Chicago. For women, intimacy leads to more satisfaction in their roles as wife and mother. For men, being able to be close with people creates confidence and resiliency that lets them go out and conquer the world.

21. Wild thing. Men's preferred home activity is sex, while women's is spending time with the family (number two for men), according to surveys by R. H. Bruskin Market Research and Speigel.

22. Doctored facts. Men exercise more strenuously than women do, but they also smoke and drink more, finds a study at Pennsylvania State University. Women know more about nutrition, and they get more eye exams and dental and blood pressure checkups.

23. Everyone out of the pool. According to a Gallup survey, the most popular sport for men is fishing. Women's most popular sport? Swimming.

24. The pits. It may be indelicate to say so, but women's are smellier. Men perspire more heavily on their chests and women more heavily under their arms.

25. Wake up, Irene. Studies suggest that men spend more time in shallow sleep as they get older and may even start skipping deep sleep altogether, says Arthur Spielman, Ph.D., director of the Insomnia Treatment Center in New York. For unknown reasons, aging doesn't affect women's sleep as much.

26. Left leanings. Most men put their pants on left leg first, while the majority of women start with the right leg.

27. Eat and run. Men are 31 percent more likely to choose foods and beverages to improve athletic performance but find it more difficult to eat healthful snacks than women, according to a poll by HealthFocus, a Pennsylvania food consulting firm.

28. A man's heart. Men have double the risk of heart disease that women have, a tendency that some researchers attribute to the male hormone, testosterone. Evidently the hormone triggers the production of cholesterol. Men also have higher blood levels of stress hormones, which cause the heart to beat harder and blood pressure to rise.

29. Bully for you. A Norwegian study found that most school bullies are male, and that while the tendency of boys to bully rose with age, in girls, it dropped. Researchers conclude aggression is partly biological in nature and, again, testosterone may be the spur.

30. Dieting. One out of three women diet, compared with one out of five men.

—Marc Bonanni and Susan A. Nastasee

Bridging the Gap

Just how wide is the chasm between men and women? This list may hold some surprises for you.

Our goal in compiling the following list was never to dispute the existence of a gender gap. There's always been one, and always will be. Rather, we wanted to get a fix on just how wide that chasm is these days.

Pretty wide indeed, it turns out. For starters, with all the talk of equality, men are still society's leaders. The CEOs of 497 of the Fortune 500 companies are male. For their part, women continue to outlive men by an average of seven years.

Just what you expected? Perhaps. However, many of the statistics we uncovered defy conventional wisdom. For example, despite decades of "Just wait until your father gets home" stereotypes on television, it turns out that only 30 percent of men spank their children, while 71 percent of women do. And only 23 percent of women, but 35 percent of men, admit they've used a headache as an excuse to avoid sex. Read on for more surprises.

Average number of doctor's visits a man makes per year: 4.5
Average number of doctor's visits a woman makes per year: 6.2

Heaviest weight lifted overhead by a man: 560 pounds
Heaviest weight lifted overhead by a woman: 286 pounds

Fastest mile run by a man: 3:46.32
Fastest mile run by a woman: 4:15.61

Chance that a man will be struck by lightning: 1 in 1,800,000
Chance that a woman will be struck by lightning: 1 in 8,000,000

Chance that a man will become a high-ranking executive: 1 in 11
Chance that a woman will become a high-ranking executive: 1 in 20

Percentage of men who are college graduates: 22
Percentage of women who are college graduates: 16

Percentage of violent-crime victims who are men: 62
Percentage of violent-crime victims who are women: 38

Number of men on Death Row: 2,211
Number of women on Death Row: 33

Nobel Prizes awarded to men: 588
Nobel Prizes awarded to women: 24

Male members of American Mensa, the U.S. high-I.Q. society:
    35,139
Female members of American Mensa: 19,011

Chance that a man talks to himself: 1 in 12
Chance that a woman talks to herself: 1 in 7

Percentage of men who would like to lose weight: 42
Percentage of women who would like to lose weight: 62

Percentage of men who like the way they look in the nude: 68
Percentage of women who like the way they look in the nude: 22

Percentage of men who snore: 53
Percentage of women who snore: 23

Chance that a man is color-blind: 1 in 25
Chance that a woman is color-blind: 1 in 50,000

Percentage of men who say they find a woman's face to be her
    most attractive feature: 27
Percentage of women who say they find a man's face to be his
    most attractive feature: 55

Chance that your best friend fantasizes about your wife: 1 in 2.5
Chance that your best friend's wife fantasizes about you: 1 in 6.6

Percentage of married men who have had an extramarital
    affair: 37
Percentage of married women who have had an extramarital
    affair: 29

Success rate, in a study, when men tested the pickup line "Hi" on
    women in a bar: 71 percent
Success rate when women tested the pickup line "Hi" on men:
    100 percent

Percentage of men who enjoyed the first time they made love: 86
Percentage of women who enjoyed the first time they made
    love: 41

Average number of intercourse positions a man knows: 14
Average number of intercourse positions a woman knows: 9

Percentage of men who prefer sex with the lights on: 45
Percentage of women who prefer sex with the lights on: 17

—*Melissa Gotthardt*

Don't Go Away Mad

The secret to getting along better with women may well lie in learning how to argue with them. Here are the rules every man should know.

Why can't men and women get along better? The prevailing view these days is that men are terrible at talking out their feelings. However, in studies of why couples split up, University of Denver psychologist and family therapist Howard Markman, Ph.D., found that hiding from emotions wasn't the problem. "Men do just as well as women at communication and intimacy," he says.

The real issue, Dr. Markman discovered, is that we are so uneasy about arguing with the women we love that we often withdraw at the first sign of conflict. "Women mistake that for rejection, and often incorrectly believe that we don't want to express our feelings or aren't even capable of it," he says.

Many relationships collapse under the weight of all that miscommunication, in large part because couples aren't skilled enough at constructive arguing. But learning to argue better is a skill like any other. According to Dr. Markman, people can learn how to have better relationships. He and his colleagues have developed and tested a method he calls "Fighting for Your Marriage" to train people to better handle their disputes. We asked him to explain his methods and the thinking behind them.

Q. Why do men find arguing so distasteful?

A. First of all, we like to have rules for handling stress and conflict. In situations where men do really well—business, sports, war—disagreements are handled by following rules. It's something we're trained to do starting at an early age. Ever since preschool, for example, my son Mathew has loved kickball, which is guided by rules and relies on outside arbitrators such as adults or older kids to settle disputes. In fact, even in warfare, there's a general convention for fighting. But there's no set of rules for couples to handle their disputes.

Second, a number of studies have shown that arguing actually feels physically different for men. It's more upsetting and unpleasant. Blood pressure, heart rate and all the other indications of how we respond to stress rise faster, higher and for a longer period in men. Without rules, men may feel more helpless in the face of a dispute, and sometimes just don't know what to do.

Q. What happens in a typical fight?

A. It often starts with the woman bringing up an issue: "We have a problem with money" or "You don't talk to me" or "We need to spend more time together." Often, the man perceives what she's saying much more negatively than she's intending. Next, the guy—even if he's staying involved in the discussion—often signals in some way that he's not interested in talking. He withdraws, perhaps by turning away from her, rolling his eyes and saying to himself, "Here we go again." The woman then pursues the discussion, often in an increasingly negative way, and the man withdraws more. In our research labs, we make videotapes of couples doing this.

In many cases, the man may try to cut off the discussion by agreeing with her prematurely—"Yeah, you're right, so tell me what to do and I'll do it." This buries the issue and it will likely come back to haunt the couple later on. Or, sometimes, he may come back with something negative such as "You're always attacking me. You're just like your mother," and all of a sudden they're really off into an increasingly negative cycle of attacks and counterattacks.

Q. It sounds as though men have good reason to think talking only leads to fights.

A. That's an interesting point, because it may become a self-fulfilling prophesy. The more a man fears fighting, the more he withdraws and actually increases the chance of a fight occurring. The other part of the picture is that the woman usually misreads his withdrawal as something negative about her. This gets her angry or hurt—exactly what he's trying to avoid. Often the man then focuses on her anger, which in turn only upsets her more. Instead, he should focus on how he can avoid withdrawing. Watch out for blaming your partner. This is a danger sign. Both people actually feed the escalation process. The sad part is that they each start out wanting to do something positive.

Q. You've said that you can predict with 90 percent accuracy whether a marriage will succeed. What are the clues signaling that a relationship is at risk for problems?

A. There are three major danger signs. The first is that the man routinely withdraws from conversation.

The second is rapid escalation during arguments—for example, fights that erupt out of nowhere over embarrassingly trivial things. When disagreements don't get resolved, there's a buildup of negative emotions that explode like volcanoes. Some eruptions are predictable and some are not.

The third danger sign is invalidation. That's where, for example, the guy spends all Sunday cleaning up the house instead of watching football, and when his wife gets home she says, "You were going to clean the house, but the kitchen is still a mess." He feels he has been unfairly attacked, which is very damaging. If this happens a lot, he eventually starts feeling he's being attacked even when he's not.

Now, your relationship isn't necessarily doomed if you face these situations once in a while. But unhappy couples (and those at risk for unhappiness) find these patterns happening more frequently than couples destined for success.

Q. How can couples resolve their differences better?

A. One key is to establish certain ground rules for discussing issues in a way that isn't threatening. First, you need to set up a regular time every week where both of you can bring up your concerns. Make sure you won't be interrupted—let the answering machine pick up calls while you're meeting, have the TV off and the kids asleep. The idea is that if you talk about issues in a structured, controlled way, they won't come up so often at other times, and when they do you'll be able to discuss them more calmly.

Q. This sounds as if you're making an appointment to have a fight.

A. The way to keep that from happening is for both people to use what we call the speaker/listener technique, in which one person talks and the other just takes the words in. The speaker should keep the message brief and to the point, limiting comments to the issue at hand. Then every few minutes, you reverse roles and the other person gets the floor.

Being the listener is the harder job. You need to make sure you're understanding what your partner is saying without defending yourself, agreeing or disagreeing. It's not a point/counterpoint debate, but an attempt to see things from the other person's perspective. One important technique is to stop the speaker every 20 or 30 seconds and paraphrase what she's said to make sure that what you're hearing is what she means.

This method counters the three destructive patterns I mentioned earlier. It stops the man from withdrawing by keeping both partners active in the discussion, it confines escalation by allowing issues to be discussed in a controlled manner and it prevents invalidation because one partner is continually affirming the other by paraphrasing. Any couple following this procedure should be able to have a constructive discussion about anything in their relationship. However, like any other skill, it takes practice.

Q. What are the potholes to look out for?

A. A lot of people prematurely try to solve disputes before both partners hear each other out. This is particularly true for men, who tend to want to fix problems, to "patch things up." Often, the issues don't actually need to be solved; 70 percent of the time, people just want to be heard.

Q. Are you suggesting we should avoid coming up with solutions for our problems?

A. The time and place for problem solving is after the issues are on the table. At first, you may want to postpone talking about possible solutions until the next meeting. But as couples get better at this process, they can ultimately talk about an issue and solve it within 20 minutes or a half hour.

Q. What if you don't have anything you care to discuss?

A. You simply yield the floor. But there are ways of helping couples identify the ongoing issues in their relationships. We have simple forms people can fill out that are like a checklist of common areas of contention, such as money, sex, communication, kids, careers. There are always things to talk about.

If neither person really has anything to discuss, keep your appointment as a special time for just the two of you. Go for a walk, give each other back rubs, make love. It can be a lot of fun, although you shouldn't try to combine these talks with fun things. For example, don't go out for dinner to have your meeting. We find that when couples are doing something clearly defined as fun, they ban sensitive issues from their conversation. For a lot of couples, the best place to meet is the kitchen, over a cup of coffee.

Q. Is it possible to develop better relationship skills outside the relationship?

A. It's generally easier to take what works well in an intimate setting and apply it outside the home than it is to take things that work well at the office, for example, and use them at home. A man is particularly likely to say, "Well, I'm good at this stuff at work, but not at home, so it must be her fault," which is not very successful thinking on his part. But it's not his fault, either. For example, on the job, men are highly reinforced for problem solving, but not for listening. I often see airline pilots, lawyers, engineers and other professionals who are very successful in their careers, and may even see themselves as good communicators, but who become totally frustrated when they faithfully try applying what they do at work to their personal relationships. Also, we don't want our airline pilots to spend time talking about their feelings while they're landing a plane.

Q. What other guidelines do you suggest?

A. Establish a rule that either of the partners can bring up an issue at any time. You don't have to wait for the weekly meeting, and in fact you should try to deal with issues as soon as they arise. But the person who's listening has the right to say, "This isn't a good time." It's then the listener's responsibility to make sure that the issue gets discussed, preferably within 24 hours.

Q. So, what is the payoff of using these methods?

A. In our studies, we've seen divorce rates reduced by 50 percent, and higher rates of marital happiness.

Because of AIDS and the growing perception that divorce isn't working as an option, people are now more motivated to have solid relationships with one partner. At the same time, it's harder for couples today because the roles for men and women are more equal than they were in the past. Suddenly, everything is negotiable, and there's a premium on problem-solving skills, which most people sorely lack.

You're in a relationship to have fun, to have a friend, to make love, maybe to have kids. You're not in it because you like conflict. But some conflict is inevitable. If you learn how to handle it, you'll be able to enjoy those other things to the fullest.

—Richard Laliberte

PART 6

Sex

Long-Distance Lust

A long and happy life is a long and sexy life. Here's rock-solid advice on how to boost your sex drive at any age.

When you're 20 and you have trouble getting an erection, you can shrug it off as nerves or too much beer at the frat party. When you're 40 and the same thing happens, you start to wonder if it's signaling the end of a long and rewarding sexual career. You've heard the conventional wisdom: After 40, or even during one's 30s, sex drive heads south; erections start balking, and when they rise, they're only flying at half-mast. In other words, like many a man's hair, male sexuality recedes and eventually disappears.

The conventional wisdom is wrong. Aging does bring some sexual changes, but they're minor. The fact is, sexual vitality is largely independent of age. If you want a great love life at 45 or 55, or 85 for that matter, you can have it.

Here's another common myth we're going to blow out of the water: Men don't peak sexually at 18. What the research actually shows, according to the *Kinsey Institute New Report on Sex,* is only that men's sexual *daydreaming* peaks then. When asked how often they had sexual thoughts, young men ages 12 to 19 said they think about sex every five minutes; men in their 40s said they had sexual thoughts about every half hour. So guys in their 40s who think about sex 30 times a day aren't exactly shriveling up. And one reason teens daydream about sex so much (besides having so much time to kill in math class) is that they're less likely to *have* sex routinely available to them.

And when we talk about staying sexually active, we're not just talking about baby boomers here. A University of Chicago survey of 6,000 married couples over 60 showed that 37 percent had sex at least once a week.

But don't men lose their erections as they grow older? There's another myth in serious need of debunking. Experts estimate that only about 5 percent of 40-year-olds suffer erection problems; at 65, the figure is 15 to 25 percent. Most of it is caused not by sexual difficulties but rather by medical conditions such as diabetes and by drug treatment of other nonsexual conditions. "Erection problems," says John C. Beck, M.D., a gerontologist at the University of California, "are not a natural part of aging."

Sex Is Lifelong

Evolution endowed us with a lifelong capacity to reproduce. But, of course, we're not 18 forever. What really happens sexually as we age? For otherwise healthy men, surprisingly little. Aging brings a slow decline in production of testosterone, the hormone responsible for men's sex drive. But most men produce much more of this hormone than they need, anyway. Even late in life, when testosterone levels are on the low side, they're still usually within the normal range. And the hardware itself remains virtually unchanged. "If I showed you a photograph of a man's erection at 20 and at 80, you would not be able to tell the difference," says urologist Dudley Seth Danoff, M.D., author of the book *Superpotency*.

So now you know the good news. Does that mean you're guaranteed to stay potent until they carry you away? Not necessarily. But there are a number of things you can do to ensure that your sex life stays vital and vigorous.

Relax, then get excited. Too much stress is hell on the libido. In an admittedly bizarre study at the University of Utah, psychologists wired the penises of 54 volunteers, ages 21 to 46, with an instrument that measures erection, then showed them X-rated videos and recorded their arousal levels. Some of the volunteers were then wired with a new fake electrode and were told that at some point during a repeat showing of the sex videos, they would receive a painful, but harmless, electrical shock. Guess what happened. Right: Arousal plunged 35 percent in those expecting a shock.

Stress works its sexual mischief in two ways. It triggers the fight-or-flight reflex, which sends blood away from the central body (and penis) out to the limbs to supply the muscles involved in self-defense and escape. It also stimulates the secretion of cortisol, a natural chemical that suppresses production of sex hormones. "The message is 'Relax,'" says Louanne Cole, Ph.D., a San Francisco sex therapist. "You'll feel more aroused and your erections will stand up better." To relax your way into great lovemaking, try a hot bath or shower beforehand—either solo or with your partner. In addition to setting the stage for good sex, hot baths increase blood flow into the penis.

Simmer all day and cook all night. Try a technique called "simmering," suggests sex therapist Bernie Zilbergeld, Ph.D. Most men have moments of sexual arousal several times a day: the beauty in the Corvette on the way to work, the cute waitress at lunch, the sexy ad in a magazine and the phone call from the client with that Kathleen Turner voice. You can hold on to those zingy moments by simmering, which Zilbergeld describes in his book *The New Male Sexuality*. Whenever you have a sexual feeling toward a woman, go ahead and focus on it for a few moments. Let yourself fantasize about her, guilt-free. Then let go of the thought. An hour later, return to it and relive it. Continue replaying your fantasies every few hours, but as you get ready to go home, substitute your steady for your fantasy ladies. Simmering keeps feelings of arousal bubbling away until you and your lover are ready to make them boil.

Try a natural aphrodisiac. For centuries, oysters have had a reputation for being aphrodisiacs. While oysters contain no magic sex-enhancing ingredient, they *are* high in the mineral zinc, an important component of semen and the prostate gland. Men with moderate to severe zinc deficiencies may suffer impaired libido and low sperm counts, according to Sheldon Saul Hendler, M.D., Ph.D., assistant clinical professor of medicine at the University of California, San Diego. Other foods rich in zinc include lean meats, seafood, whole-grain products and wheat germ. No other specific foods hold a promise of sexual ecstasy, but one diet does. It's the same low-fat, low-cholesterol diet the American Heart Association (AHA) recommends to prevent heart attack. In addition to keeping off extra pounds, the AHA diet may prevent the clogging of the arteries that supply blood to both the heart and the penis. A low-fat diet might help sex drive in another way as well. A recent study by endocrinologist A. Wayne Meikle, M.D., of the University of Utah showed that four hours after consuming a high-fat meal, participants' testosterone levels dropped 30 percent, possibly enough in some cases to dampen sex drive.

Stay sensitive. One significant age-related change in the penis is a gradual loss of sensitivity to touch, because as the years pass, the nerves in the penis lose some ability to transmit stimulation to the brain. One way to compensate, says sexual medicine specialist Theresa Crenshaw, M.D., of the Crenshaw Clinic in San Diego, is to use a sexual lubricant. In recent years, science has produced several new ones that feel slicker and less messy than the longtime commercial leader, K-Y jelly. Check in your pharmacy for Probe, Astroglide and other inventively named sexual lubricants.

Get aerobic, get erotic. Want to work up more sexual energy at any age? Then work up a good sweat. Recently, University of California researchers studied 95 out-of-shape men, average age 47. Seventeen took little strolls for one hour three days a week, while 78 got sweaty in more strenuous aerobic workouts.

After nine months, the strollers reported no change in sexual desire or activity and an increase in sex problems. But the aerobic group reported a jump in sexual desire, a 30 percent increase in frequency of intercourse, fewer sex problems and more pleasure from orgasm.

Harvard anthropologist Philip Whitten, Ph.D., came to the same conclusion in a study of male swimmers ages 40 to 69. Those in their 40s reported sex about seven times a month—almost twice a week. That's about 40 percent more sex than the average man in his 40s has, according to *The Janus Report on Sexual Behavior.*

Be strong where it counts. Any moderate regular exercise adds to sexual longevity, but one particular exercise actually boosts the intensity of orgasm. Known as Kegels after Arnold Kegel, M.D., the doctor who popularized them, this intimate workout strengthens the pubococcygeus (or PC) muscle that runs from the base of the penis to the tailbone. To do a Kegel, squeeze the same muscles you would use to stop the flow of urine. Do a set of ten contractions several times a day. Within a few weeks, you should notice that your orgasms feel more intense and pleasurable.

Lose a little weight. Ronette L. Kolotkin, Ph.D., of the Duke University Diet and Fitness Center, surveyed the effects of weight loss on 64 participants, average age mid-40s. The study is still in progress, but her preliminary results are revealing: "Moderate weight loss (10 to 30 pounds) significantly improved the sexual desire and feelings of attractiveness," Kolotkin says.

Coffee keeps things hot. When researchers at the University of Michigan surveyed 744 married couples ages 60 or older, they discovered that the daily coffee drinkers among them were almost twice as likely to describe themselves as "sexually active"—62 percent, versus 38 percent of the noncoffee drinkers. Coffee-drinking men also reported fewer erection problems. The reason for the connection isn't yet understood.

Don't mix sex with these drugs. Moderate amounts of stimulants may arouse the libido, but many other drugs do the opposite, says James Goldberg, Ph.D., research director at the Damlugi Bari Clinic in San Diego, California. The main offenders are:

• Blood pressure medications, especially the so-called calcium channel blockers, such as Procardia and Calan.

• Most tranquilizers, especially Librium, but also Valium and Xanax.

• Any pain relievers containing codeine.

• Most antidepressant drugs, with the exception of some of the newer types, such as Wellbutrin.

• Anti-epileptic drugs such as Dilantin.

• Ulcer and other stomach disorder drugs such as Tagamet and Reglan.

If you experience sexual problems and are using any of these medications, consult your doctor. A lower dosage or a switch to an alternative medication may get you back in the game.

Nonprescription medications can also make your libido go slack: "If the label says 'May cause drowsiness,' it's probably a sex offender," Dr. Crenshaw says. These include many cold and flu formulas, some allergy products and motion sickness drugs.

Go easy on the booze if you want to boogie. Alcohol is probably the world's most sex-dampening drug. It may relax inhibitions, but beyond that first drink, alcohol becomes a central nervous system depressant that impairs libido, erection and sexual pleasure. A general rule is that the amount of alcohol it takes to affect your driving ability (for an average-size man, anything more than two drinks in an hour) can also affect your libido, says Dr. Goldberg.

Stand by your woman. So you're envious of your bachelor friends? Don't be. Your sex life will be a lot better if you work on tending your own garden than if you try your hand playing the field. According to *The Janus Report on Sexual Behavior,* couples are more sexually active than singles. Forty-seven percent of singles described themselves as sexually active to very sexually active. Among couples, the figure was 54 percent. And almost 60 percent of those in couples said that sex had improved after marriage.

If marriage enhances sex, divorce often crushes it. Researchers at Wayne State University in Detroit extracted data on the sex lives of 340 divorced people from a large national sample and found that over a year's time, one-quarter were celibate and only one-quarter made love more than once a week. "Divorce is depressing," says sex therapist Cole, "and depression impairs libido."

In the end, though, demography works to older men's sexual advantage. On average, women live longer than men. Not generally the best of news for us, but if we stay fit and eat right, we can reap the rewards at the end. At age 65, there are 1.25 women for every man. By age 80, women outnumber men two to one. Stay healthy and sexually active long enough, and you'll live to see what the Beach Boys discovered in Surf City—two girls for every boy.

—Michael Castleman

Female Sex Secrets

If women could give us love lessons, here are the secrets they would want to teach us first.

"This is where you put 'it' in," she said.

Twelve years ago Todd, Geoff and I were three midwesterners just out of college living in a fourth-floor walk-up on the fringes of Greenwich Village. We had moved to New York City to begin careers, and we were taking our first awkward steps in this new world. I suppose the same could be said about our first relationships with women.

One night around midnight, we got to talking about women, sex and women's bodies. In a way it was typical guy talk for men in their early twenties, except that there was a woman present, a girlfriend of Todd's. One of us had confessed to having trouble figuring women out "down there," so in service to us (and perhaps to other women) she opened a spiral-bound notebook and drew a circle, followed by three smaller circles arranged vertically inside the first one.

It was then, indicating the largest of the three inner circles, that she told us where to put it. We were transfixed. "And this is where we go to the bathroom," she continued, pointing to the circle just above it. "Because they're so close, sex, and even petting, hurts us sometimes. It's also why we get so many damn infections." We hadn't even gotten to the clitoris, when it occurred to me: If we, three college-educated adult men living in the big city, needed help with the basics of women's bodies, what about other men?

It's not that we didn't have any girlfriends of our own. After all, this was before AIDS was an issue, and we were young and single in a city teeming with available women. But as the impromptu anatomy lesson demonstrated, we had a lot to learn.

Now, in my midthirties, I'm a veteran of several long-term relationships, as well as some briefer entanglements, but I've yet to marry.

What Do Women Want in Bed?

And I still find myself asking questions. Indeed I often think that the power to read minds, were it available, would be best appreciated in the bedroom. Just imagine if each time you made love to a woman she knew exactly what you wanted as soon as, or even before, you did. And imagine that you knew exactly what she wanted. There'd be no need to ask, to take that risk of saying or doing the wrong thing.

Fortunately, as a journalist I can ask questions on the job, even the intimate questions that men often keep to themselves. But in my quest to learn more about the minds and bodies of women, I had another factor working in my favor—they wanted to talk. Like Todd's girlfriend from our Greenwich Village days, the women I interviewed about sex were delighted by the opportunity to reveal the secrets they've always wished men knew, even if they were afraid to tell them to their own lovers.

While no book or magazine article can claim to be exhaustive on so complex a topic, following are the six sexual secrets women volunteered most frequently.

1. She's starved for praise. A woman's body image can bring her more torment (or pleasure) than most men ever realize. Part of the reason is sociological: Women who subscribe to social and media norms feel compelled to look "appealing, earthy, sensual, sexual, virginal, innocent, reliable, daring, mysterious, coquettish and thin," in the words of author Susie Orbach. Countless women pursue a kind of physical perfection that is impossible to achieve. It's not surprising, perhaps, that up to 200,000 women underwent breast augmentation surgery in 1989 alone and that at least 10 million women are affected by eating disorders.

In light of this vast aesthetic uncertainty among today's women, men need to recognize that praising a lover's beauty doesn't just boost her ego, it makes her feel comfortable.

Speaking of the best lovers in her life, Judy H., a graduate student, says, "It's not just what they did, but how relaxed they made me feel. They made me confident about my body. And they made me feel really loved."

"The sounds of silence make it real hard to relax," adds Pat H., 27, a single artist from New England. "Talking is important, even if it's just someone saying, 'I really find you attractive' or 'You're so soft.' Or if he says my name. I want to see his tender side."

"When I'm having sex with someone, I'm aware of where his eyes go, and whether or not he wants the lights off," says Sharon L., 31, once divorced, from Providence, Rhode Island. "If a man gets up and turns the lights off, I take that to mean he doesn't want to see my body. As sexually confident as I am, it's not the same with my body. If a man isn't responsive, I withdraw. It's that simple.

"I think it's harder being a woman," she adds, "because we're worrying about breast size, fat thighs, stomach rolls and wrinkles. You want them to make you feel that none of it matters. I think in our hearts, everyone wants to be told she's beautiful."

2. Be twice as gentle as you think you should be. Sometimes, even as we strive to please, we men can come on too strong. One of the most important leaps a man can make sexually is to realize that what he feels below his waist is not what his partner feels. In fact, women may feel very little through the walls of the vagina most of the time, because the nerve cells located along the vaginal walls are not all that plentiful. (And the clitoris, as we all know, the nerve center of female pleasure, is located outside the vagina.)

So what may be most pleasurable for a man, the deep, thrusting, in-and-out motions of intercourse, may provide very little sexual satisfaction for a woman. She may prefer woman-on-top positions, in which she can more carefully direct the thrusts toward stimulating her clitoris. Or she may prefer shallow penetration, and positions in which the tip of the penis rides along the outer edges of the vagina, where the most excitation, nerve response and swelling naturally occurs.

"I think the biggest mistake men make is that they touch you as hard as they want you to touch them," says Judy H. "It just doesn't work that way."

3. Learn to linger. This may be fundamental. Think of Mae West, arch-sex symbol of the 1930s, who sang the praises of "A Guy What Takes His Time": "I don't like a big commotion/I'm a demon for slow motion" were just a few of the lyrics that shocked many people by revealing the long-suppressed truth about female sexuality. Even in our relatively enlightened time, speed remains an issue. For while the occasional "quickie" can be as thrilling for our mates as it is for us, women usually find that rushed sex is bad sex.

The reason? Beyond emotional needs, women simply take longer than men to climax.

The experience of Ann M., 22, of Madison, Wisconsin, is typical in this sense. She had been sexually active for six years before she actually began to enjoy intercourse in a relationship that made her feel physically comfortable and "adult," orgasm and all.

Speaking of the man who opened her eyes to the erotic possibilities, she says, "It really helped that he was so patient."

Judy H. made a similar discovery. "I never had an orgasm till I was 20, even though I'd already slept with a lot of people," she says. The change came with a boyfriend, John, who patiently spent enough time with her to make her relax completely. For the first time she didn't feel as though she had to rush, even though she took a lot longer to climax than her partner.

In short, Ann and Judy found lovers who, in the words of Mae West, "would condescend to linger awhile." And for them, that made all the difference.

4. Discover her secret pleasures. Compared with the male body, which betrays its arousal even when clothed, the female body retains an air of subtlety, even mystery. Witness the confusion surrounding the clitoris—among women as well as men.

A number of women I spoke to admitted not knowing even where to find their clitorises until more experienced, or possibly better read, boyfriends showed them.

"When I started dating in the early 1950s, almost none of my sexual partners seemed to know what or where a clitoris was," says Alice W., 48, a married writer from the Midwest. "Sometimes I thought I didn't have one or it was in the wrong place."

When a woman is aroused, a number of things normally happen. She experiences clitoral swelling, a flush about the chest and neck, sweating and nipple erection. When doctors or sexologists speak of "clitoral erection," they're referring to the head of the clitoris and the immediate surrounding area, which is composed of erectile tissue. Surrounding this sensitive tissue are nerve endings that, in the right hands (and with the right stimulation), can greatly increase a woman's pleasure.

It's also worth knowing that as orgasm approaches, the clitoris momentarily shrinks out of sight, burrowing back beneath its hood. This may confuse many men, who see it as a sign of sexual turnoff when in fact, at this stage, it's a sign of intense arousal.

5. If you question, so will she. It's here that my wish for mind-reading powers returns with renewed urgency. For while it's obvious enough that women appreciate a lover who attends to their needs, questions such as "Does this feel good?" are not always welcome.

Teresa R., a single 25-year-old from the Midwest, says that sometimes plain talk works in bed, sometimes not. "Women today are not as afraid to say what does and does not feel good," she says. "But when I tell my boyfriend something doesn't feel good—when he puts his finger in a certain place in my vagina, for example—it makes me feel like I'm at the gynecologist."

Karla D., a 28-year-old secretary from Philadelphia, says she wishes men were more adventurous with her body. But there are times when she feels like having sex without needing to "teach" a partner in bed. Recently, when one man said, "Karla, tell me what makes you feel wonderful," she was glad he asked, but at the same time wished he didn't have to. When told that that kind of question is tough for the average man to ask, she says, "Trying to come up with an answer is hard, too. I mean, I'm not trying to make it scientific."

In her latest book, *Women on Top,* Nancy Friday picks up on this theme: "Men might learn if women told them exactly what they wanted. But women hate giving instructions to the man, telling him what to do, what it is they want; getting involved in their own seduction makes them too responsible, breaks the mood of being swept away."

So where does that leave us poor men who aim to please but don't always know how? Perhaps Elyse A., 26, of New York has the right idea. "It would help if men knew a woman has more nerve endings on the outside of her body than on the inside," she says. "They can learn it by sensing what the other person is doing while they're touching. You don't always have to explain it."

Judy H. recalls that her boyfriend John changed her usually detached reaction to receiving oral sex by exploring her genitals carefully and by watching—feeling—her body's reactions to his motions, and by spending enough time with her that she felt she could relax completely.

In sex, then, the best communication may be nonverbal. A man needs to read a woman's body rather than always rely on her to put her wishes into words.

6. Once you know the rules, break them. While learning all the ins and outs of intercourse can do a lot for one's sex life, there is a subtle danger of becoming obsessed with performance and technique, of trying too hard.

"Some men think, 'I'll do this for ten minutes, then that for ten minutes, then roll her over,'" says Eleanor H., 34, a legal assistant from South Carolina. "Are they reading this in a magazine? They want their partner to go back to her friends and say 'John really knew what to do.'"

"I've had two guys who have been amazing," says Terri D., 26, once engaged but never married. "They taught me that having sex isn't an exercise, that there's so much potential. And yet some men look at it as piecework, step-by-step, then orgasm, then you go to sleep."

"I guess at 22 I had a list of 'performing' things," says Sandi L., 28, a physical therapist from Cleveland. "Now I don't give a hoot about them. There's no list. Whatever happens that day happens. And it's more enjoyable in that there's no A, then B, then C. It never gets boring."

Needless to say, when men are excessively concerned with performance, they tend to spoil the fun for themselves as well as for their partner. "Accused of being selfish, men are not really selfish enough," says Paul Pearsall, Ph.D., in his bestseller, *Super Marital Sex*. "For they are too busy trying to do instead of be and experience. Love becomes a product they try to 'make.'"

While being spontaneous carries a certain amount of risk, it can also lead to the greatest satisfaction. Knowledge is better than ignorance. But sometimes the thrill of discovery is best left to the participants.

—Curtis Pesman

Shape Up Your Sex Life

How to keep that sex machine of yours mechanically sound for a long, long time.

Joseph Khoury runs a couple of miles every morning, eats a low-fat diet and swims for half an hour most days to relieve stress. While it's a routine that will certainly keep his heart strong and his mind clear, he has another motive, something most guys in their midthirties don't think about, but should.

"I've never had a problem with erectile function, and I don't plan on having one either, because I'm doing something about it now," says Khoury. Now it's only fair to point out here that Khoury is not your average health-minded guy. He's a urologist at Georgetown University Medical Center in Washington, D.C. Which is to say he has studied the equipment responsible for producing erections and he has observed what happens when men take care of the equipment... and what happens when they don't.

Few of us are as forward-thinking as Dr. Khoury. We take a lot of things for granted in life, especially when we're young and seemingly omnipotent. Right through our twenties, we didn't have to work out as often to stay muscular. We ate whatever we wanted and didn't gain weight. And we never thought twice about getting an erection. If anything was a problem in that department, it was getting one too often. "All you needed was a girl to walk by in a tight sweater," says John Mulcahy, M.D., a professor of urology at the Indiana University Medical Center in Indianapolis. "And at night, the penis would get as hard as a piece of plastic pipe."

But now that many of us have passed the age of 30, business might not be as usual. We already know that as our metabolism slows down, it takes more time in the gym to maintain our muscle tone. Most of us can't indulge in certain foods the way we used to without bulging at the waistline.

137

And guess what? "Whenever things start to go to pot in your body, the erection will be no exception," says Dr. Mulcahy. The basic science behind erectile function has only emerged in the past decade or so. And while the research is revealing that a complex interaction of hormones and brain chemicals are necessary, "all it really is, is blood flow," says Dr. Mulcahy.

What the Penis Needs

Just as the heart needs open blood vessels to receive an adequate supply of oxygen, the penis requires an open pathway to receive blood for an erection. And just as fat in the bloodstream can build blockages in the arteries of the heart, so can it build blockages in the arteries of the penis.

Studies of artery plaques show that they are present in our bodies as early as our teens. But as a rule they don't affect the function of the heart until after age 50, when heart attack rates escalate in men. However, because some blood vessels to the penis are narrower, they may show signs of unhealthy living earlier.

According to the experts, the average man in his thirties will begin to notice that his erections aren't quite as firm as they used to be and that they don't respond to those tight sweaters as rapidly. And thanks to the added stress we carry as we climb the career ladder and begin raising families, the odds are greater that moments will occur when our penises say no when our brains say yes.

It doesn't have to be that way. In fact, if you look at studies of men who stay fit and trim and know how to relieve stress, you see little if any decline in erectile function through middle age. "Theoretically, there is no reason for your potency to change as you age," says Dr. Khoury, who knows men in their eighties who still have sex three times a week. The one thing they have in common: They took care of themselves better than most men. "I believe this could be a big incentive for keeping fit," says Dr. Mulcahy.

Where to start? According to the experts, if you smoke, quitting tops the list of advice for improving sexual fitness. Cigarette smoking accelerates the formation of blockages in the heart's arteries, and there's every reason to believe that it does the same to the vessels that supply blood to the penis. In fact, smoking is now considered a major factor in erectile dysfunction, with the first signs of harm appearing by age 40.

Besides leading to plaque buildup along artery walls, nicotine in tobacco is also a blood vessel constrictor. That means each puff makes it more difficult for blood to get to the penis when it's stimulated. When men stop smoking, Dr. Mulcahy says, most will get firmer erections. It's a subtle improvement, and some smokers don't realize they had a problem until they quit.

Aerobic Sex

Second on the list is to develop an aerobic exercise routine. The more fit you become as a result of exercise, the more sex you'll have and the better it will be, says a study published in the *Archives of Sexual Behavior*. They're not just talking *perceived* better. They're talking more orgasms. In the study, 78 healthy but inactive men began aerobic exercise three to five days a week, for an hour each time. Another control group simply walked at a moderate pace three to five days a week. During the study, each man kept a diary of sexual activity. The results showed that the sex lives of the aerobic exercisers significantly improved. The more they exercised, the more and better sex they had. Meanwhile, the sex lives of the walkers changed very little.

It doesn't matter which type of aerobic exercise you choose, as long as you do it a minimum of two to three times each week and stick with it for at least 20 minutes per session. Running and rowing are both good choices.

When it comes to diet, the bottom line is limiting your fat intake. Again the logic goes that what's good for the arteries supplying blood flow to the heart will also be good for those supplying blood to the penis.

How much fat you can safely consume is still under debate. While the American Heart Association recommends less than 30 percent of daily calorie intake from fat for the average man, Dr. Khoury argues that a "high-potency" diet ought to be approximately 20 percent fat.

Limiting fat in your diet also reduces weight gain, and according to Dr. Mulcahy, excess pounds can actually make critical inches of the penis disappear. Informal studies he has done of obese men show that—up to a point—a man will regain one inch of his penis for every 35 pounds of weight lost. Not a bad incentive for someone who is really heavy. But more practically, keeping your weight down will reduce the risk of high blood pressure and diabetes, both of which impair the ability to have an erection. Keeping blood pressure normal also means avoiding antihypertension drugs, which can cause impotence.

Stress Leaves You Limp

While not smoking, staying fit and eating right will avert problems down the road, mental stress is probably the greatest cause of erection trouble now, says Jack Jaffe, M.D., director of the Potency Recovery Center in Van Nuys, California. "In our society we're under stress throughout the entire day, and our sex life tends to suffer later in the evening," he says.

It was not easy to find men willing to recount a story about such an experience. But after much wheedling, a friend I'll call Frank, who lives in a town I'll call Baltimore, allowed as how he once had a problem in bed. It was at a time in his life when the stress was thick indeed. He'd been wrapped up in a bitter separation from his wife for months, bickering over money and custody of their child. After the divorce was final, he was amazed to meet a woman interested in a no-strings-attached arrangement. Following several weeks of getting to know each other, the time came for a particularly romantic evening. But during the hours before his date, Frank says he engaged in a rancid argument with his ex-wife over an upcoming weekend visit with his three-year-old son. The conversation stayed in his mind the entire evening.

"My girlfriend was dressed to kill and she was in the mood," he says. "But all I could think about was how to strangle my ex-wife. Nothing was happening below the belt."

Dr. Mulcahy says it's common for stress to interfere with the ability to raise an erection. But he also says it's important to let the incident drop. Guys get into trouble when they worry that something terrible is wrong with the equipment and that the problem will recur. Then they get a recycling and magnification of the problem, which leads to performance anxiety. And, the human brain being the practical joker that it is, if you expect trouble, you'll often find it.

The one thing you don't want to do is drink alcohol to relieve stress. Shakespeare probably said it best in *Macbeth* when he described alcohol as that which "provokes the desire, but . . . takes away the performance." For a more contemporary model, we have Jim Morrison, whose well-documented whiskey binges led him to write a poem titled, "Lament for the Death of My C—k."

Alcohol is a depressant that slows down reflexes, including sexual ones. Besides impairing immediate performance, alcohol when consumed excessively for too long can have a direct effect on the testicles, decreasing production of testosterone, upsetting the delicate balance of hormones and brain chemicals required to make an erection.

Act Your Age

Finally, however strong your potency is, there's no point in trying to compete with the 20-year-old you. You and your partner are bound to have a bit less spontaneity in your sex life than you had back then, if only because you have more on your mind, greater responsibilities, richer interests and a fuller schedule. Dr. Jaffe says the way to avoid psychological problems here that could interfere with your performance is not to wait for the magic moment. "You've got to make it happen," he says. "That may mean setting a date, sitting down to discuss what your needs are, whatever it takes."

Bottom line: A man's got to put some work into maintaining his youthful potency. But this ought not to be a burden. Dr. Khoury sees it all as a kind of symphony. Staying fit makes you feel good and look good. Eating right and properly relieving stress gives you energy: "It all coincides really quite elegantly. You run, you eat a good diet, you get a good body image and you keep your mind at ease—all of that ties into your sexuality," says Dr. Khoury. "It really is something worth working for."

—Tim Friend

Spread Pleasure

Take off your clothes together and rediscover the joys of the soft, caring touch. Learn the forgotten art of sensual massage.

"With a warm, quiet place and a bottle of scented oil, you can spread pleasure over every inch of your partner's body," says Gordon Inkeles, bestselling author of *The Art of Sensual Massage.*

What a pity that we so seldom do it.

Even people who love each other and have been happily married for years tend to forget 95 percent of the vast and varied vocabulary of touch. After a few years of a relationship, the way we touch each other tends to be reduced to one of two things: We do it either in a completely sexless, perfunctory way (a peck on the cheek, a pat on the back) or in a way that is as sexual as you can get. Often, when a man touches his mate at all, it's basically a way of asking a question: "Do you want to have sex?" First comes the touch, then the kiss, then a fast-forward to orgasm.

Even when we get sexual, the places that we touch each other tend to be limited to a couple of square inches of skin the dimensions of an airmail envelope. Whole kingdoms of the body, and of sensuous pleasure, go unnoticed. Says Inkeles: "It's entirely possible that a woman who's been married for years has never been touched behind the knee, or between the toes, by another adult since childhood." Our whole culture, in fact, is so starved for touch that sometimes people will have sex when all they really want is the feel and warmth of skin against skin.

Never Too Late

But it's never too late to learn the exquisite pleasures of touch and rediscover each other in the process.

It's called *massage.*

Don't be intimidated by the word. There are types of massage that require lots of training and maybe even a few courses in human physiology, but that's not what we're talking about here. We're talking about simply using touch to give your partner pleasure and then unashamedly *receive* it (which is also the goal of satisfying sex). That kind of touch doesn't take any particular training at all, although it does require that you care for each other.

Massage is a potent sex enhancer, says Inkeles, because it induces deep relaxation and rapidly dissipates the negative effects of stress. People tend to have sex as a way of relieving physical tension. But a far better approach is to slip into a state of deep relaxation *first,* through sensuous massage, and then make love.

For one thing, the ascent to orgasm (which, momentarily, involves extreme body tension) is much more dramatic if you first go *down* into a state of deep relaxation, rather than starting from a state of semiaroused agitation, says Martha Brown, a registered massage therapist in Charlottesville, Virginia.

"The biggest obstacle to great sex," Inkeles adds, "is stress." And sensual massage is one of the oldest and most reliable stress reducers in the world.

Massage, whether or not it's overtly sexual, is also just a delightful way to express affection. It's a way to explore the forgotten frontiers of your partner's body and in the process vastly expand your repertoire of touch. And it's a way of finding out what makes your lover feel good and what doesn't.

The How-To Part

Preparing for a sensuous massage is like setting the mood for love. It doesn't have to be terribly involved. Just find a space in your life where you're sure you won't be interrupted—the bedroom is fine. Take the phone off the hook. Lock the door. Put the clock in the drawer and forget about time. Don't focus on giving your lover a massage for any particular amount of time—just do it for as long as it feels good.

Massage oils are nice because they feel great and tend to make the skin more sensitive to touch. You can buy expensive massage oils, but ordinary safflower oil works fine, as does coconut oil. It's best to warm the oil a little before use. Try putting it in a plastic squeeze bottle for convenience. Instead of oil, some people like to use cornstarch, which is so silky to the touch it almost feels wet.

Other things to remember:

• People tend to touch each other during massage in the same way *they* like to be touched. The result: Men tend to massage women too firmly. The solution: Just keep asking for feedback. "How does this feel?" "Should I bear down harder?" "Is that too soft?" The only unforgivable sin of massage is to make your partner feel uncomfortable. Says Inkeles: "One moment of pain destroys an hour of good massage."

• People tend to hold lots of tension in their faces. Try massaging the forehead, jaw muscles, temples. Use strokes that smooth out or go across the lines on the face. Another great spot to focus on: the feet.

• Women tend to hold tension in their neck and shoulders; men tend to hold it in the small of their backs, Inkeles says. Give those areas special attention.

• Any spot where the skin is thin is especially sensitive, such as around the ankles, the insides of the arms and the neck.

You really don't need any fancy equipment to give a great massage, but sometimes a vibrator can be used for spice. Try strapping the device to the back of your hand, so that your fingertips transmit the good vibrations.

Massage as Therapy

The marvelously sensuous magic of massage has not been lost on sex therapists. In fact, a form of massage has been a key part of many sex therapy programs for the past 20 years. First developed by William Masters, M.D., and Virginia Johnson, of the Masters and Johnson Institute in St. Louis, sensate focus exercises, sometimes also called nondemand pleasuring, are a way for couples in sexual distress to break free of mutually reinforcing avoidance. But even people who are not having sex troubles can use them to great effect.

Basically, nondemand pleasuring works like this: A couple gets naked together in a quiet, romantic place and takes turns caressing each other's body. (Usually, at least to begin, the couple is seated, with the receiver sitting between the giver's legs.) There's just one rule: The breasts and genitals are off-limits, and so is intercourse. That way, there is no pressure to push forward to orgasm, no pressure to achieve anything or get anywhere, no pressure to return any favors. The only place to go is into the sensuality and stillness of the present moment.

—*Stefan Bechtel*

The Fine Art of Ogling

You spot her. You give her the once-over lightly. You stare. She stares back. Now what?

Ever notice how traveling through life is a little like vacationing in Boca Raton with Zsa Zsa Gabor? You sort of hate to say anything, but the plain truth, to pretzel-wrap a metaphor, is that Life overpacks, and it's you who ends up carrying the steamer crates filled with frilly little lessons and sequin-encrusted inescapable laws. Well, here's the deal. In this little space, at least, I'm your redcap. I guess sorting out the baggage is my job, given my profound affection not just for explanation, but for pontification.

It's an easier job than most, owing to the plentiful supply of resources. In fact the best part of life is the puzzle page, figuratively speaking, where enormous weighty subjects—death, women, work, government, shoes—can be discussed with proper deliberation. Here's something, for example: What does it mean when you're ogling a woman and she catches you at it, and instead of looking away, gives you a direct stare not once but *twice?*

I call this the Rule of Double Eye Contact on a Single Ogle. Case in point: two fortysomething guys. A mall. An escalator. Two women, mid-thirties. One ogle. Two eye contacts.

The details: a sunny day, but brisk. Two friends—we'll call them Hoot and Gib—decide to meet for lunch at a downtown enclosed shopping mall. There's a quick dash into a Brooks Brothers outlet, where a suit is purchased within three minutes. Then there's lunch.

The dining area at the mall is one of those American adaptations of a Euro-trough, the standard street café. Next to the café is a descending escalator, and next to the escalator is where our two chaps encamp for a quick bite. One guy, Hoot, is married, and he has his back to the escalator. He can't see anything, girlwise. The other guy, Gib, is single, and he can see everything. The escalator practically dumps shoppers at his feet.

The conversation is a heavily fragmented one. Hoot talks about media coverage of the deficit. Gib is frequently distracted by the sudden appearance and descent of one or another metropolitan beauty. In the middle of a sentence, he suddenly clams up, raises one eyebrow in a sullen smolder, and, frankly, ogles. He's been doing this for years, of course, and his scan is a well-practiced one. The face is his screening device. Bad face, back to the deficit. Good face, go directly to the shoes and work up. He ogles like a bibliophile, like a man who knows exactly which details and nuances create desirability and which ones are fatal flaws. Hoot waits patiently for the appraisal.

Measure Yourself

The Brown Corollary: A man ogles not just to fantasize about women, but, according to writer Ian Brown, to see how he measures up as a man. Generally—and there are certainly exceptions to this corollary—he is making a precise calculation that involves this equation: Self-image divided by her beauty plus her availability equals relative worth of ogler. There are many tiny variables that can nudge the ultimate solution one way or another. For instance, you might look at a beautiful passerby and find she is almost certainly out of range of your ability to attract women. Maybe the self-image part of the equation is too low, or her beauty-plus-availability number is too high. But then you say to yourself, "Sure, that's now. But a dash of Rogaine, a few years on carrots and sprouts and a Samsonite full of C notes and she'd be at my feet." Suddenly, your projected self-image numbers rise, and you find it more and more likely that not only could she be yours (if you really wanted) but maybe you wouldn't have time for her, what with all the other women around.

But back to the Double Eye Contact on a Single Ogle rule. When a normal guy is ogling, part of what he's actually doing is just thinking about what politely might be called a relationship. But sometimes in ogling, as in all relationships, things sort of sneak up on you. For instance, after a burger-and-fries' worth of idle ogling, Gib suddenly pales. "I got eye contact," he says tensely, almost grimly. "No, wait. That's it." His voice drops to a burdened whisper. "I got double eye contact."

The sequence is this: Contact. Ignition. Liftoff. Double eye contact in response to a single, lingering ogle is a gesture of commitment more meaningful than many marriages. When a woman returns an ogle with a single glance, it can mean anything. Might mean: "What's he staring at? Is there toilet paper on my shoe?" Might mean: "Let's see what kind of jerk I'm dredging off the bottom of the gene pool today." Might mean: "Make a move and I call the cops." Hence, most men disregard the Single Glance to an Ogle response.

I See You, Too

A double glance, however, is something else. Double Eye Contact on a Single Ogle means this: "I know you're watching me and I think you're sort of marginally interesting and I think I'll see what you're made of, buster."

So. You ogle. She does a double take. Now what do you do? If you look away, too stunned or embarrassed to continue ogling, you're scrapple. A guy too cowardly to stand up for his own ogle isn't much of a man in most women's books. But if you continue to ogle in the face of a double glance, the ball's back in her court. If she looks away, no point. If she smiles, you can figure you've been asked to politely identify yourself, your motives, your marital standing. If your papers are in order, you get permission to cross the line, to go the next step. Whatever that is.

The Never-Fail Principle of Bad Timing: Women almost never return an ogle until your wife or girlfriend is looking—first at the woman, wondering who she's smiling at, and then at you when she figures it out.

Because we men ogle as a means of taking stock of ourselves, we know there's nothing intrinsically threatening about the whole activity. We don't ogle, after all, because we want to. We ogle because we have to. It's horrible sometimes. Call it ogle burden. But sometimes a man's gotta do what a man's gotta do.

To Each His Own

That's why different men ogle in different ways. Involved men out with the objects of their involvement do an indirect ogle. They look around the supermarket as if they'd never seen anything quite like it before. "Look at those lighting fixtures!" they seem to be saying. "And how about those metal shelving units!" Their necks are suddenly rubberized for such occasions, and the fact that a clearly ogle-able woman just happens to be in line of sight is pure coincidence. That way, if the woman responds to the ogle with a smile, the guy can always look at his ferocious wife and shrug. Men know they can ogle their brains out and never get so much as a notice until one fine, spring day when an ogling kind of guy and his principal sugar pie are out for a stroll. He tosses off an inconsequential ogle and presto! He gets a double—no, a triple!—take in return. Then he starts explaining.

Guys out in packs do competitive ogling. A woman walks down the street, and there's a wild pack of oglers staring at her. She nervously glances over to make sure they aren't armed oglers, and instantly every man jack claims eye contact. "She was looking at me, man," one of them says, while the others produce documentary evidence refuting the claim.

A single-man ogle is a serious thing. Women know that. That may be why they so infrequently respond.

The Law of the Knowing Glance: The glance-to-ogle scenario has many variations. One of them involves the situation reversed, where she is the ogler and you are the oglee. Women ogle as much as the next guy, by the way. Usually, they ogle other women, although since their mission in ogling is essentially fact gathering—"Why did she wear that scarf?" "You call that eyeshadow?" "Nice pumps"—it may be demeaning to ogling to call it ogling. Women sometimes ogle men. *That's* ogling. If you're on the receiving end, you might be well advised to invoke the Law of the Knowing Glance, which says an ogle is always trumped by a leer. In other words, you slowly look up and meet her gaze, while on your face you wear an expression that says, "Was that good for you?"

Now What?

This has the effect of ram-injecting the encounter and giving it a NASA-level rate of acceleration. Suddenly, you're not just two strangers exchanging ogles for gapes. You're on intimate terms, with you, Mr. Mojo, in the driver's seat. You saw her ogle and raised her an innuendo. You can't lose. If she looks away, give her five minutes, and she'll ogle again. If she smiles, you can figure your glance was good enough that you can roll over and go to sleep. Either way, you'll have this encounter in the bag, if you'll pardon the play on words.

The Obviated Ogle Injunction: An ogle is diminished by over-shadowing eccentricities. Let's say you're sitting alone in a subway car when a gaggle of art school painters' models—women who have been ogled with aesthetic passion—gets in. They're young, they're beautiful and they stare right at you. The significance of their attention all depends on why they're staring. If it's because you're wearing a Santa suit and darning your socks, all ogles are off. No return glances are scored, and your self-image numbers are expressed in negatives.

Ogle-proof women: Finally, it's good to note that there are women who are at least ogle-resistant, if not downright ogle-proof. To wit: all nuns, the Queen of England, Andrea Dworkin and Imelda Marcos.

—Denis Boyles

PART 7

Disease-Free Living

Can You Catch It?

Not all diseases are created equal. Some are more contagious than others. Knowing whether something is catching is the first step in prevention.

Some guys worry about catching a cold from the bathroom water glass and cold sores from pay phones. And who knows what microbial assassins lie in wait among those petrified globs of bubble gum stuck to the bottom of the movie seat?

We live among billions and billions of exotic bacteria, viruses, fungal spores and assorted unseen stuff. Most of these invisible neighbors are harmless, but a few can make you various degrees of sick.

The trick, of course, is to find ways to avoid the harmful bugs and to ignore the others. Doctors are learning more each day about the ways diseases are spread. Here's an updated guide to what you can and can't catch—and how best to protect yourself.

AIDS

We all know by now that AIDS is contagious, but there seems to be a lot of needless concern about getting the disease from casual contact with someone who's infected. The human immunodeficiency virus (HIV) can be transmitted through anal, vaginal or oral sex with an infected partner or by sharing drug needles with a person who has the virus. That's why those at greatest risk are intravenous drug users and people with numerous sexual partners—homosexuals and heterosexuals alike. "A high level of promiscuity just increases the risk of exposure," says Albert Balows, Ph.D., former assistant director for laboratory sciences at the Centers for Disease Control (CDC) in Atlanta.

Should the paramedic worry about mouth-to-mouth resuscitation? Should the barber toss away his brush and comb? "All we can tell them is to do as they normally would," recommends Dr. Balows. There is no evidence suggesting that AIDS can be transferred through inanimate objects. Small concentrations of the AIDS virus have been found in the saliva of infected people, but former Surgeon General C. Everett Koop, M.D., Sc.D., says that as long as no blood is present, saliva, sweat and tears pose no threat. "You won't get AIDS from a kiss," he says. Nor from insect bites.

Those who worry about getting AIDS from a blood transfusion should know that the risk of this has been greatly reduced. Blood donors are now screened for risk factors, and donated blood is tested for the AIDS antibody. You cannot become infected when you donate blood.

The surest way to avoid AIDS is to limit sex to one mutually monogamous, uninfected partner. Beyond that, a latex condom, used with a spermicide such as nonoxynol-9, is the best preventive measure.

Athlete's Foot

Contagious. But for reasons not clearly understood, some people resist the fungus that can cause the itching, burning and scaling of athlete's foot. Bacteria also play a role in bringing about peeling and blisters.

Athlete's-foot fungi thrive in a moist environment. That's why locker-room shower floors and shoes that don't let the feet breathe can be perfect breeding grounds for athlete's-foot fungi. Topical, over-the-counter antifungal ointments can be effective in banishing the fungi from between toes.

Canker Sores

Possibly contagious. The cause of these painful mouth ulcers remains a mystery. Experts theorize that they might be spread by kissing or sharing a drinking glass with someone who has a sore.

Common Cold

Highly contagious. How does that cold virus find its way from someone else's red nose to yours? Cold viruses attack the upper respiratory tract. When cold sufferers sneeze or cough, they spray extremely fine droplets of virus-bearing mucus and saliva into their environment. "There's no such thing as a dry sneeze," says Dr. Albert Balows. "The smaller the droplets are, the greater the trajectory they have and the longer they float in air."

Why do we repeatedly get sick some years? Because there are so many different cold-causing viruses, explains Dr. Balows. "A person can develop a cold from virus number one and, following recovery, may develop an immunity that will protect that person for some time. But it doesn't give him a nickel's worth of protection from virus number two."

If you don't have a cold, staying away from those who do is the best prevention, although that's easier said than done. In the meantime, the search for a cold cure—a search some researchers consider an impossible dream—goes on. Among the proposed remedies: interferon, a natural antiviral substance produced in the body, now being reproduced in quantity in the laboratory.

Dermatitis

Contagious. *Pseudomonas aeruginosa* is the full name for the bacterium that flourishes in inadequately chlorinated hot tubs. It causes skin rashes known as "hot-tub dermatitis" as well as swimmer's ear and urinary tract infections. Although such cases are rare, it's also possible to catch pneumonia by inhaling superfine water droplets contaminated with this bacterium. In general, the warm, moist environment of the spa is a disease bug's playground.

Eczema

Not contagious. The cause of this itchy skin disease remains unknown, but you can't catch it from someone else. Remedies—not cures—range from topical steroids to cold cloths to diet therapy to a change of climate.

Hepatitis A

Contagious. The primary mode of transmission is the fecal-oral route—typically when an infected food handler prepares food without first washing his hands. To lessen the likelihood of contracting hepatitis A while dining out, make sure your food is adequately cooked. Washing your own hands frequently reduces the risk of picking up the virus from hand shaking.

Hepatitis B

Highly contagious. Hepatitis B is usually far more serious—and more common—than hepatitis A. The virus is spread via any exchange of bodily fluids, including blood transfusions, kissing, and anal, oral or vaginal intercourse. Symptoms usually include joint pain and jaundice, and sufferers are at risk of being afflicted with chronic hepatitis, cirrhosis of the liver and liver cancer.

Herpes Simplex

Both oral and vaginal herpes can be transmitted through sex—vaginal, oral or anal—and skin-to-skin contact such as kissing. The virus is most readily (but not exclusively) transmitted when sores are present. In simulated testing, intact latex condoms provided an effective physical barrier against genital herpes during sexual intercourse, but doctors still recommend abstinence when herpes sores are present. That's because the condom only covers the shaft of the penis—sometimes sores can form in other areas of the genital region.

Can you catch herpes from a toilet seat in a public rest room? The odds are extremely low, say the experts. The virus can survive on a plastic toilet seat for about an hour, but for others to contract it, the skin of their thighs or buttocks would probably have to be broken. According to the CDC, there are no documented cases of anyone being infected via a toilet seat. The same goes for public telephones, hot tubs and swimming pools.

For now at least, there is no cure for herpes. But the prescription drug acyclovir is effective (in pill form) in reducing pain and shortening the period of the virus's activity. (Acyclovir topical ointment is not so effective.) Progress is being made on a vaccine that would prevent herpes infection as well as recurrences in those already infected.

Jock Itch

Contagious. Jock itch is caused by the same fungus that causes athlete's foot, so it also thrives under warm, moist conditions. Keeping the infected area dry and using an antifungal topical ointment is usually enough to eradicate the fungus.

Strep Throat

Contagious. In rare cases, this bacterial infection—characterized by a sore, red throat and high temperature—can lead to rheumatic fever. It's transmitted by direct or by indirect (e.g., sneezing) personal contact. A less-publicized mode of transmission is inadequately refrigerated food. The adaptable bacteria are also known to cause skin infections in athletes who participate in contact sports such as wrestling and rugby.

Syphilis

Contagious and still quite prevalent. The disease has four increasingly nasty stages. The first usually consists of painless sores in the genital area and on the lips. The second stage is characterized by a measleslike rash that can cover the entire body. In these stages, syphilis is highly contagious and can be spread via sexual contact, kissing or any contact with the sores or rash. If syphilis spreads to the eye, it can lead to blindness.

In the third stage, the virus appears to retreat into dormancy, where it can rest for years. Syphilis is not thought to be contagious in this stage. The last stage may not appear for more than 15 years after initial symptoms have disappeared. At this point, the disease is much less contagious, but it can be fatal: The bacteria can invade and damage any part of the body, including the heart, brain and nervous system.

In the first three stages, syphilis can be cured effectively with antibiotics such as penicillin and tetracycline. In the fourth stage, it may be more resistant to antibiotics and never completely cured. Although a latex condom may provide protection against syphilis if the sores are covered, it's best to abstain from sexual contact if one partner is infected.

Trench Mouth

Not contagious. Although the bacteria that cause trench mouth are thought to be present in many people, only a small percentage of those people suffer with the periodic mouth ulcers and pain. Outbreaks are usually associated with stress or illness.

Warts

Contagious. You can't catch warts from a frog, but you can get them from another person. Warts are caused by a virus, which enters the skin of the susceptible person through a cut or scratch. Before you can catch warts, your immune system defenses must be lowered, generally through illness. Wart viruses can be picked up either by direct contact or indirectly in moist environments, such as showers or swimming pools.

—Jeff Meade

Be Your Body's Best Friend

How to give the slip to ten common health problems, including athlete's foot, heartburn and ingrown toenails.

Backache, heartburn, food poisoning, ingrown toenails—they probably won't kill you, but if you've ever had a bad case, you won't want to repeat the schooling. Fortunately, doctors and scientists have come up with some pretty good ways to bypass many everyday health hassles. So learn your lessons the *easy* way. Here's how to avoid ten common bummers.

Athlete's Foot

Even if you're an armchair athlete, you're not immune to this fungus. Athlete's foot is a fungal infection that produces burning pain, itching, cracked, peeling skin, bleeding and blisters. Balmy climates, such as you find inside sweaty shoes, are what makes this fungus thrive. Once you have it, it takes about four weeks to medicate it away. Here's how not to catch it in the first place.

Don't be a Shoeless Joe. Damp floors can spread athlete's foot from one health-club member to another. Wear flip-flops in the locker room, shower room or spa. After showers, dry your feet thoroughly. (Use a hair dryer on them if you want, but don't let anyone catch you doing it, or you may never live it down.)

When it's hot, hit the spot. Use Tinactin, Halotex, Desenex or another athlete's-foot product daily to weekly in hot weather, even if you don't have an active case. Spray the insides of your shoes as well.

Change your shoes. Don't wear the same pair of shoes two days in a row, advises Chicago podiatrist Dean S. Stern, D.P.M. He says it takes at least a day for shoes to dry out thoroughly. If your feet sweat heavily, you may need to change your socks three or four times a day.

Back Pain

Sooner or later, nearly one-half of the guys with blue-collar jobs and more than one-third of those with desk jobs will end up having back troubles. These preventive measures can help keep your back younger and trouble-free.

Get up, stand up. "Just stand up for five minutes every hour, and I guarantee your back will feel better," says physical therapist Phil Dunphy. "Stand when you talk on the phone, or take a short break to walk around at regular intervals while you're at work."

Or have a seat. Conversely, if your job requires long periods of standing, have a seat every 15 minutes or so, says Suzanne Rodgers, author of *Working with Backache*. The ideal chair, according to the American Medical Association (AMA), has a tiltable back support, adjustable height, and a contoured seat edge that supports three-fourths of your thighs but doesn't cut into the backs of your knees. Adjust the height so you can sit with your feet flat on the floor and your knees level with or slightly higher than your hips. Keep your work surface at elbow height.

Don't read flat writing. Prop your book at a 20-degree angle in front of you, or hold it parallel to your face.

Invest in a good mattress. Hard beds are best and water beds are second best for back pain sufferers because they both evenly distribute weight, according to tests done by the Division of Orthopedics and Rehabilitation at the University of California, San Diego.

Don't offer to help your friends move. Lifting puts more stress on the spine than any other action, especially if it's done wrong. If you must move big stuff, stand close to the object, bend your knees while keeping your back vertical, grasp the object and hold it as close as you can as you *slowly* stand using your leg muscles. Leaning out and over to lift something, as from the trunk of a car, places an enormous load on your spine and is a notorious slayer of backs. Lay those jumbo bags of dog food on the back seat. Anytime you can use a hand dolly to move heavy objects, do it. Otherwise, push, pull or slide them.

Food Poisoning

You get food poisoning two ways: by eating food that actually contains poison, produced by the bacteria growing in it (botulism and staphylococcal food poisoning are this type); or by picking up a bug from food contaminated with organisms (such as salmonella bacteria) that multiply in the body.

Botulism is rare but deadly, killing one-third of the 10 to 15 people who get it each year in the United States. About 75 percent of the cases of botulism are traced to improperly home-canned foods. Here's how to avoid botulism.

When in doubt, toss it out. Scientists estimate that one cupful of the pure botulism toxin could kill all the people on earth. The point is, don't even taste food from a swollen can or from a jar with a swollen lid. Ditto for food that is foamy, moldy, or has a bad odor. Dispose of the food in such a way that there is no chance it will be eaten by street people or by animals.

Unlike botulism, salmonella infection is common: It makes more than five million Americans a year bow to the porcelain goddess. Abdominal pain, diarrhea and fever are other lowlights of salmonellosis. Avoiding salmonella infection is relatively simple.

Keep your bird cool. Store raw poultry in the refrigerator down low, where it can't drip onto other foods. Rinse it thoroughly before cooking, and dispose of juices from the package. Frozen poultry should be thawed overnight in the refrigerator or in a plastic bag under *cold* water, not just left out.

Don't egg yourself into trouble. Eggs are another potential source of trouble. Skip the Caesar salads and soft-boiled or over-easy eggs. Eggs need to be cooked at least three minutes at 140°F to be safe. Use only uncracked eggs and keep them stored no longer than five weeks.

Stow stuff right. Improper storage temperature causes the most cases of food-borne illness, and many occur at picnics. Bear in mind: Bacteria thrive at temperatures between 40° and 150°F. "There is one very simple prevention rule—keep food *hot* or keep it *cold*," says Edmund Zottola, Ph.D., professor of food microbiology at the University of Minnesota.

And cook it well. Unless the inside of your food reaches 165°F or hotter, salmonella could survive. Considering that a study at Iowa State University found salmonella in 41 percent of packaged cut-up chickens, you'd better cook that bird until the inside is white. If you're barbecuing, microwave the pieces for about half the time you would in a microwave recipe, and then throw them on the flames.

Soup cold? Send it back. Restaurants account for about one-half the outbreaks in the United States. Check that the food is well cooked and that hot foods are hot and cold foods are cold. One Food and Drug Administration (FDA) honcho says, "I won't eat warm tuna salad, and I send back soups that are lukewarm."

Sandwich seminar. When you brown-bag it, pack frozen sandwiches, recommends the University of Oklahoma Health Sciences Center. They will thaw by lunchtime. Simple sandwiches freeze best, such as those made with peanut butter, sliced meat or poultry or with mixtures that do not contain mayonnaise, mayonnaise-type salad dressings or hard-cooked eggs. Carry lettuce, tomatoes and dressing to add to sandwiches later.

If possible, keep your sandwich in a refrigerator at work until lunchtime. Some sandwich fillings made with meat, poultry, fish or egg can spoil if kept at room temperature for more than two hours.

Headaches

Nine out of ten headaches are caused by muscle tension, according to the National Headache Foundation. Tension headaches usually produce a generalized pain, like a steel band is being tightened around your skull.

Researchers aren't sure what causes the other two types of head pain—migraines and cluster headaches. An estimated five million American men suffer migraines, which typically produce severe, one-sided, throbbing pain, often accompanied by nausea.

While three times as many women suffer migraines, men are cursed with 90 percent of all cluster headaches. Sufferers say these feel like a red-hot poker is trying to get out through the backs of your eyes. These headaches may occur every day for weeks or even months. Men who get them are typically heavy smokers, says Seymour Solomon, M.D., a headache specialist at Montefiore Medical Center in New York.

You're in the best position to recognize what habits and factors bring on your headaches—and perhaps what you can do to prevent them.

Know your danger foods. For some men, it's milk. Others get killer headaches from the monosodium glutamate (MSG) in Chinese food. An amino acid called tyramine, found in nuts, aged cheeses and chocolate, socks it to others.

Watch the weenies. Pass on the mustard *and* the hot dog. The nitrites in cured meats, including bacon, bologna and some ham, can dilate blood vessels and bring on major head pain, says Houston's

Ninan Mathew, M.D., president of the American Association for the Study of Headache.

Don't sleep through breakfast. Headaches can be brought on by low blood sugar from skipping meals. "A lot of patients get migraines on weekends because they sleep through their normal breakfast time," says Seymour Diamond, M.D., of the Diamond Headache Clinic in Chicago. "It's better to get up, eat, then go back to bed."

Stay loose; sit straight. Working in awkward positions can cause the muscles in your neck to contract and trigger a tension headache, says Dr. Diamond. Check yourself for signs of tightening up—clenched teeth, clenched fists, shoulders up around your ears.

Reach for a rub. Press both thumbs under the bony ridge at the base of the skull where the neck muscles attach. Keep up medium pressure for a few seconds, then release. Don't press too hard, and don't rock or rotate your thumbs. In this way, cover the whole ridge horizontally in a two-inch-wide band. When you find a hot spot, repeat the thumb-pressure treatment several times.

No strain, no pain. Squinting in the sun or continuous staring at a video display terminal can cause tension headaches. "Take regular breaks from the computer screen and wear sunglasses outdoors," Dr. Diamond advises.

Heartburn

Its telltale signs are smoldering pain beneath your breastbone and a sharp, acrid taste in the back of your mouth. The trouble is brought on by a backwash of stomach acid and acid-soaked food sloshing up into the esophagus. A protective lining enables the stomach to withstand its own acid—including the same hydrochloric acid you watched burn a hole in your high school chemistry lab bench—but the unprotected esophagus becomes inflamed and painful. You usually feel the scorching near the base of your chest, but you could get a burning sensation as high as the back of your throat.

Fortunately, you aren't doomed to continue these slow burns. Doctors know what can cause stomach acid to back up. Change your diet and your ways, and you can extinguish the flames.

Miss the bloat. Overeating is often to blame for getting burned because it puts too much pressure on the esophageal sphincter, the "door" at the entrance of the stomach. This muscle normally relaxes only to let food *in;* but when your stomach is bloated, the pressure can force food or acid back through it and into your esophagus, says gastroenterologist Frank Moses, M.D., of Walter Reed Army Medical Center in Washington, D.C.

Also, go easy on acidic fruits and vegetables like grapefruits and tomatoes. That goes double for spicy-hot foods—a Gallup Poll found that Mexican cuisine is tops for giving people heartburn, followed by Italian food and pizza.

Don't carbo-load. Carbonated drinks like beer, soda, champagne and sparkling mineral water can increase stomach pressure, triggering heartburn.

Don't leave the door open to trouble. Avoid cigarettes, alcohol, coffee, chocolate and sedatives. These can relax the muscle door, leaving it slack enough for stomach lava to erupt into the esophagus.

Don't snack at 10:00 P.M., let alone midnight. If you're prone to heartburn, don't eat anything two hours before going to bed. Stomach acid production peaks in the first couple of hours after a meal, and lying down makes you more susceptible to problems.

Hemorrhoids

How do you find the hemorrhoid creams at the pharmacy? Head for the aisle full of pained-looking men walking very carefully. Hemorrhoids—swollen, sometimes protruding blood veins of the anus—are a real pain for eight out of ten of us. They're partly hereditary and partly caused by diet and bad bathroom habits. Here's how to avoid the agony.

Go easy. If it's news to you that defecating is not supposed to be a grunting, arduous task, you probably already have hemorrhoids. Straining engorges the veins in the rectum, and hard stools scrape the swollen area, causing more trouble.

Drink fluids, eat fiber. This reduces your chances of constipation and straining on the toilet, says Phoenix rectal surgeon Edmund Leff, M.D.

Lighten up on the salt. Excess salt retains fluids in the circulatory system that can cause bulging of the anal veins.

Ingrown Toenails

It seems like a puny problem until you get one. Then it seems like the lightning rod of hell. Here's how to keep on believing it's no big deal.

Avoid pointed or tight shoes. Ingrown toenails occur when a nail—usually on the big toe—grows or is pushed into the soft skin alongside it. Certain shoes will do that. Opt for wide-toed shoes that don't fit too snugly, says Manhattan podiatrist Suzanne Levine, D.P.M.

Don't try shortcuts. Leave your toenails long enough to protect the toe from pressure and friction. To cut them, soften the nails in warm, soapy water, then cut straight across with a sturdy, sharp, straight-edged clipper. Never cut your nails in a rounded shape so that the leading edge curves down into the skin at the sides. Always leave the outside edges of the nail parallel with the skin.

Smooth over your mistakes. If you accidentally cut or break a nail too short, carefully smooth it at the edges with an emery board so that no sharp points are left to dig into the skin.

Insomnia

Difficulty falling asleep ranks right behind the common cold, stomach problems and headaches as a reason that people visit doctors. Here are some commonsense approaches on how to put insomnia to bed.

Stick to a schedule. Try to go to bed and to get up at the same time each day so you can set your system's inner clock, says Merrill Mitler, Ph.D., director of research for the Division of Sleep Medicine at the Scripps Clinic in California. Don't sleep in too late on Saturday and Sunday. If you do, you may have trouble falling asleep Sunday night.

Set aside some quiet time. An hour or so before going to bed, reflect on the day's activities and clear your mind of the distractions and problems that might keep you awake once you pull up the covers, says David Neubauer, M.D., of the Johns Hopkins University Sleep Disorders Center.

Don't turn your bed into a horizontal office. Use your bedroom only for sleep and sex. Don't watch TV, read, argue, talk on the phone or catch up on paperwork in the sack.

Practice relaxation. Here's an easy technique: Slow down your breathing, and imagine air moving slowly in and out of your body while you breathe from your diaphragm. Do this a few times during the day so it's easy to do before you go to sleep.

Motion Sickness

The water is blue, the boat is white and you're green from seasickness. At first you're afraid you're going to die. After a couple of hours, you're afraid that you're *not* going to.

Motion sickness—be it from a boat, plane, car or camel ride—occurs when your brain gets confused between motion your inner ears sense and motion your eyes see, explains Horst Konrad, M.D., an ear, nose and throat specialist at the Southern Illinois University School of Medicine. Once the dizziness, sweating and nausea begin, motion sickness is as hard to hold back as a cresting wave. Better to steer clear.

Score some Scōp. A prescription drug, Transderm Scōp, comes in a dime-sized patch that you stick behind your ear. It releases sickness-quelling medicine into your skin for up to three days.

Press your luck. The Sea-Band, a woven elastic band worn on each wrist, contains a small plastic button that presses an acupressure point on the inside wrist, which reportedly prevents motion sickness. It's available at some pharmacies and marine shops for about $9.

Go gingerly. Powdered ginger prevents motion sickness better than Dramamine, according to a study at Brigham Young University. You can buy ginger capsules at most health-food stores. Or you can dissolve ¼ teaspoon of ginger from your spice rack in hot water or fruit juice and drink it before you travel.

Put up a good front. A cabin in the middle of a large ship does noticeably less rolling and pitching. In a car or bus, sit up front and focus on the road ahead as if you were driving. If you must read, slouch down in the seat and hold the reading material close to eye level to block out your side vision of the scenery rushing by.

Traveler's Diarrhea

Also known by a slew of ethnic slurs, it's caused by foreign strains of bacteria that normally live in your intestines and aid with digestion. These strains give you diarrhea by producing a toxin that prevents your bowels from absorbing water from fluids and foods—extra water that has to come out somehow. Okay, no more. Here's how to give it a wide berth.

Don't try everything on the menu. Avoid uncooked vegetables and fruits you can't peel, undercooked meat, raw shellfish, ice cubes and cocktails mixed with anything but bottled water (contrary to popular belief, the alcohol won't kill the bug).

Turn off the tap. When possible, stick to bottled water for drinking. Boiling water for three to five minutes purifies it, as do iodine droplets or tablets. (You can buy these at most camping stores. Follow the instructions.)

Drink orange juice or colas. Acidic liquids can help keep down the bacteria count in your gut.

Buy some trip therapy. Drink lots of acidophilus milk and eat yogurt. These foods provide a healthy level of beneficial bacteria in your colon that can help ward off a bacterial invasion. (Frozen yogurt may not work, since much of it contains no active yogurt culture.) You can buy capsules containing acidophilus and take them during the trip.

—Richard Stevens

Significant Symptoms

Forget about laughing through your discomfort. There's no gain in some pains. If you've got one of these 25, take it to the doctor—now!

We men are no strangers to pain. In fact, statistics show we are far more likely than women to be victims of chest, back, abdominal and sports-related pain. Doctors say the majority of our aches and pains are best treated with rest, a couple of aspirin, an antacid or an ice pack. But, being doctors, they like to remind us that there are some pains we need their help with.

Usually those things are . . . well, painfully obvious. "If you feel like you've been hit by a sledgehammer, then that's a good sign that you better get to a doctor," says William Ruderman, M.D., chairman of the Department of Gastroenterology at the Cleveland Clinic-Florida.

But sometimes even light taps can be a warning sign of something serious. Appendicitis, for example, usually starts with a dull ache below the navel before it intensifies. And even mild chest discomfort can sometimes be associated with heart problems.

Here's a rundown of pains you should never ignore.

Head

• A headache that's accompanied by a stiff neck, lethargy, sensitivity to light or sound, nausea or vomiting. "Eighty-five to 90 percent of all headaches don't require medical attention, but when the pain persists for more than a day, recurs frequently or is very severe or associated with telltale symptoms, then it's time to consult a physician," says Richard Lederman, M.D., Ph.D., staff neurologist at the Cleveland Clinic Foundation.

Possible problems: Encephalitis, meningitis, tumor.

• Any head pain associated with an injury or trauma that left you disoriented or unconscious. "It's not uncommon for a person to get right up after being knocked out, only to have problems arise down the road," says Lyle Micheli, M.D., associate professor of orthopedics at Harvard University and past president of the American College of Sports Medicine. "Getting checked out right away can minimize the damage."

Possible problems: Concussion, skull fracture.

Ears

• Ache in one or both ears, accompanied by hearing loss or discharge. The tricky part is that many times people feel better the minute their ears start to drain, according to Jerome Goldstein, M.D., executive vice-president of the American Academy of Otolaryngology–Head and Neck Surgery. "But the draining is *not* a sign that things are taking care of themselves."

Possible problems: Infection, ruptured eardrum, damage to bones or nerves of inner ear.

• Severe pain, especially if associated with difficulty swallowing or breathing, or accompanied by fever and chills.

Possible problems: Infection of ears or throat or tumor in the throat or mouth.

• Ringing that won't go away.

Possible problems: Wax buildup, high or low blood pressure, drug allergy, Meniere's disease (a disorder caused by damage to the delicate structures deep inside the ear).

Eyes

• Pain in one or both eyes, lasting more than half an hour or accompanied by blurred or impaired vision or extreme sensitivity to light.
Possible problems: Infection, glaucoma, corneal scratch.

Neck

• Sore throat that gets progressively worse and makes swallowing or breathing difficult, especially if accompanied by tenderness in the neck or a fever lasting more than 48 hours. "Sore throats are usually part of the common cold, but when they start getting worse after several days or they make swallowing difficult, it's time for a doctor to have a look," says Dr. Goldstein.
Possible problems: Infection of throat, such as strep throat or epiglottitis (inflammation of the epiglottis).

Chest

• Sudden, severe pain that lasts more than five minutes; pain that gets worse with exertion, is accompanied by a tightening or pressure in the chest and shortness of breath, or radiates to the jaw, neck or arms.
Possible problems: Heart attack, angina, inflammation or infection of heart muscle.

Abdomen

• Severe pain that doesn't abate within an hour and isn't relieved by antacids. Tenderness around the site of the pain. Accompanying recurrent diarrhea or flulike symptoms such as fever, chills, nausea or vomiting.
Possible problems: Appendicitis, diverticulitis (infection of the wall of the colon or the area around the colon), gallstones, intestinal obstruction.

• Less severe, persistent ache lasting more than a few days and accompanied by flulike symptoms, weight loss, diarrhea or rectal bleeding.
Possible problems: Peptic ulcer, diverticulitis or a bowel infection.

• Sharp, constant stabbing on right side below the ribs, accompanied by flulike symptoms. May also be accompanied by jaundice (yellowing of the eyes and skin), light stools or dark urine.

Possible problem: Gallstone disease.

• Mild discomfort in right upper abdomen (under ribs) with prolonged illness and fatigue. May also be accompanied by jaundice and sometimes itching all over.

Possible problem: Hepatitis.

Back

• Pain that comes on suddenly following an injury to the back or neck—especially when accompanied by loss of bladder or bowel control, numbness, tingling or difficulty moving any limb.

Possible problems: Fractured vertebrae, ruptured or herniated disk.

• Stabbing pain in the lower back or buttocks that shoots down the outside of one or both legs, especially if it's accompanied by numbness in the legs.

Possible problems: Ruptured or herniated disk, fractured vertebrae.

• Dull ache in the lower back that gets progressively worse and may be accompanied by a burning sensation during urination, along with chills, fever or other flulike symptoms.

Possible problem: Kidney infection.

Genitals

• Stabbing pain in one or both testicles, often radiating to the groin and lower back. It may come and go or be accompanied by fever. "Don't be lulled into not seeing a doctor if the pain goes away temporarily," cautions J. Francois Eid, M.D., a urologist at New York Hospital–Cornell Medical Center.

Possible problem: Kidney stones.

• Pain in one or both testicles that lasts for more than a few hours—especially if accompanied by a red, inflamed scrotum and flulike symptoms.

Possible problem: Epididymitis, an inflammation of the epididymis, the coiled passageway leading from the testis, in which sperm is produced.

• Severe pain that comes on rapidly, occurs in only one testicle and radiates to the groin and lower abdomen. "This needs immediate attention to prevent the possibility of losing the testicle," says Dr. Eid.

Possible problem: Testicular torsion, a condition in which the testicle twists on itself, cutting off its blood supply.

• Ache or burning that occurs during urination or intercourse, especially if accompanied by an unusual discharge or blood. "One incident of bleeding or unusual discharge merits a trip to the doctor," advises Dr. Eid.

Possible problems: Bladder infection, prostate inflammation, sexually transmitted disease.

• Testicle that's tender to the touch or feels harder than usual or uneven.

Possible problem: Testicular cancer, which is 90 percent curable if discovered early.

Skin

• Any sore that doesn't heal within a week, bleeds, changes color, is multicolored or has irregular borders.

Possible problem: Skin cancer.

• Pain from a sting or bite that's accompanied by progressive swelling, difficulty breathing, fever, nausea or vomiting.

Possible problems: Severe allergic reaction to an insect's sting or venom, which can sometimes be fatal.

Bones, Joints and Muscles

• Severe pain accompanied by a heavy swelling, loss of normal motion, black-and-blue discoloration or a misshaping of the limb. "Even a trained eye may not always be able to tell if a bone is broken without an x-ray," comments Dr. Micheli.

Possible problems: Fracture; severe sprain; torn muscle, ligament or tendon.

• Extreme pain in a joint, especially if accompanied by fever or rash. "Joint injuries are usually more severe than muscle or tendon injuries, and these frequently require attention," says Peter Bruno, M.D., internist for the New York Knicks.

Possible problems: Infection, fracture, torn ligament or cartilage.

• Severe pain at the base of either calf, accompanied by the inability to rise up onto your toes.

Possible problem: Severely strained or ruptured Achilles tendon.

• Nagging pain that's intensified over the course of a week or two. "Be especially wary of an overuse injury if the pain gets worse or comes on earlier each time you exercise," says Dr. Micheli.

Possible problems: Stress fracture, muscle strain or tear, tendinitis.

—Dan Bensimhon

Get It Down, Keep It Down

16 off-the-cuff tips for keeping your blood pressure down where it belongs—all day.

A while ago, I went to my doctor for a complete physical. I knew it was going to take some time, so I allocated a full hour. (Ha!) The receptionist took my name and pointed to a vacant chair. I picked up a month-old issue of *Time* magazine and sat down to wait. I finished the magazine, then another. The receptionist pretended I wasn't there. When my entire hour was almost up, I was finally escorted into a back room and told to strip to my shorts. Now, with no magazines to read and a cold draft blowing on my legs, I waited some more.

Some time later, the doctor breezed in. "How are you doing?" he asked, getting down to business by strapping a blood pressure cuff around my arm. "Fine," I said through clenched teeth, although what I really wanted to say was, "How would you be doing if some arrogant jerk kept you waiting more than a hour for an appointment that was scheduled months ago?"

"Hmmm," he muttered to himself as he took my blood pressure reading. "Do you use a lot of salt?"

No, I don't use a lot of salt. And I don't smoke. And never before, or since, has my blood pressure reading been that high. What I experienced that day is known as a *spike,* a short-term jump in blood pressure. Spikes can be caused by a multitude of things, including being pissed off.

A surge here or there is not dangerous for a healthy person. "But," says Kenneth H. Cooper, M.D., president and founder of the Aerobics Research Center in Dallas, "in people with underlying hypertension, coronary artery disease or some weakness in vessels, excessive spikes throughout the day may become a problem." In fact, they may make the condition worse and could trigger a heart attack.

In contrast to spikes are the factors that push blood pressure up more slowly, but keep it high—things like eating salty foods, drinking to excess and smoking. Ultimately you want to avoid both kinds of high blood pressure, because men with hypertension are seven times more likely to have a stroke and four times more likely to have a heart attack.

Controlling high blood pressure without drugs isn't easy, and you shouldn't even try until you've discussed it with your doctor (who I hope won't *give* you high blood pressure like mine did). But it's a worthy effort. Drugs prescribed to treat hypertension are strong medicine, with common side effects such as impotence, depression and chronic fatigue.

These tips aren't meant to be a complete program for lowering blood pressure, but they are proven techniques that can help. Work as many as you can into your life and you should see some very positive results.

1. Tell the truth. As I discovered in my doctor's examining room, blood pressure tends to spike when you lie. That's because fibbing requires your brain to work harder, according to David Robertson, M.D., director of the Clinical Research Center at the Vanderbilt University School of Medicine. "When you lie, you have to think about the truth, then manufacture something different from the truth." It's hard work. Stressful, too, since there's the potential for being found out.

2. If you don't drink coffee, don't start. For some reason caffeine tends to boost blood pressure in people who don't drink it very often. In one study, bus drivers were given the equivalent of one to two cups of coffee. Those who rarely drank coffee had a surge of over five points in their blood pressure readings.

3. Rent *Annie Hall*. Or any other movie that makes you laugh. A good chuckle relaxes your body and may release endorphins, the brain's natural stress-reducing chemicals.

4. Get a dog. Having a pet is a calming influence. The minute you start talking to or petting any animal, blood pressure drops a little and stays down as long as you maintain the contact. One study even found that people who watched tropical fish in an aquarium had a measurable, if temporary, dip in blood pressure.

5. Don't shout. Simply avoiding loud, aggressive tones may help keep blood pressure from spiking during an argument. In a study conducted by Aron Siegman, Ph.D., professor of psychology at the University of Maryland, increasing speech rate and voice volume were linked to increasing blood pressure. "If you change your speech pattern so you speak slowly and softly, even when you're angry, you will feel less angry," says Dr. Siegman.

6. Eat in Italian restaurants. In European studies, 47 patients with mildly high blood pressure who received a daily 600-milligram dose of garlic powder (roughly three to four cloves' worth) showed an average drop in blood pressure of around 11 percent.

7. Order the fish. Omega-3 fatty acids, found in ocean fish such as mackerel, tuna and salmon, may help counteract hypertension, according to a number of studies. In one report, 16 subjects taking fish-oil supplements showed as much as a four-point drop in blood pressure. Researchers still need to establish a stronger link between fish oil and blood pressure. Meanwhile, experts recommend eating fish at least twice a week.

8. *And* the broccoli. Boosting your fiber intake is one of the most important dietary changes you can make to lower blood pressure. Experts believe that increasing your fiber to 20 grams per day not only helps lower blood pressure but also reduces cholesterol. Fruits, vegetables, whole grains and legumes all head the list of good fiber bets. If you can't get enough in your diet, ask your doctor about taking regular doses of a fiber drink such as Metamucil.

BLOOD PRESSURE PRIMER: WHAT THE NUMBERS MEAN

Blood pressure readings are actually a double measurement of the force of the blood against arterial walls. You need two measurements so you can tell how much pressure builds up in the arteries both as the heart beats and between beats. The high number gives a sense of the pumping force of the heart. The lower number indicates flexibility and clogging in the arteries.

The reading is usually taken by wrapping an inflatable cuff around the upper part of your arm. Air is pumped into the cuff until circulation is cut off. At this point, when a stethoscope is placed over the artery in your arm, nothing can be heard. Then the air is slowly let out of the cuff until you can hear blood begin to flow through again. This is your systolic pressure, the high number in your reading, and it's expressed in how high it would send a column of mercury in a tube. A reading of 120 millimeters is considered normal.

As air continues to be let out of the cuff, the pressure of the cuff becomes so low that the sound of the blood surging against partially closed artery walls disappears. This is the diastolic pressure, the low number. A normal reading is 80 millimeters.

Readings above 140/90 indicate hypertension. In effect, it's a sign that the heart is working extra hard to get blood through the circulatory system, because of narrow or inflexible arteries or both. Over a period of time, an overworked heart becomes enlarged and less efficient. And the added pressure damages arterial walls, leading to scarring and hardening of these vessels.

9. Get into training. There's evidence that moderate weight training may be as effective as medication in lowering blood pressure. However, since lifting weights can also temporarily raise blood pressure, if you have high blood pressure or a heart problem, see a doctor before starting a program.

10. Run, walk or bike. Regular aerobic exercise not only lowers blood pressure, but it can help you prevent it in the first place. "People in good shape are simply less likely to develop hypertension," says Dr. Cooper, who observed this phenomenon while monitoring the effects of exercise in 4,600 people over five years. Aerobic exercise also reduces the magnitude of short-term pressure spikes, minimizing their harm to the blood vessels.

11. Shed that potbelly. Researchers have reported dramatic drops in blood pressure after men got rid of their spare tires. In one study, 60 percent of hypertensive patients who lost weight controlled their blood pressure so successfully that they were able to stop taking medication.

12. Take C and see. Two separate studies have found that people with the highest levels of vitamin C had the lowest blood pressure—and vice versa. To add vitamin C to your diet, eat more citrus fruits, green peppers, broccoli, tomatoes, strawberries and cantaloupes. You can also take vitamin C supplements.

Other research suggests that potassium brings blood pressure numbers down. Experts recommend getting at least 2,000 milligrams of this mineral each day. One baked potato contains 844 milligrams; one banana contains 451. Other good sources include dried apricots, lima beans, Swiss chard, skim milk, oranges and chicken breast.

13. Bone up on calcium. Several studies have uncovered a link between low calcium intake and high blood pressure. And there's further evidence that upping calcium intake to normal levels can bring high blood pressure down for some individuals. If you have high blood pressure, it's a good idea to make sure you're getting at least the men's RDA (Recommended Dietary Allowance) of 800 milligrams, equal to a little less than three cups of skim milk.

14. Don't let the job kill you. In an experiment, employees ranging from stockbrokers to sanitation workers estimated the on-the-job stress they felt. They then donned portable monitors to gauge their blood pressure as they worked. Those who reported high job stress were three times as likely to have high blood pressure as those who didn't report a lot of stress.

You owe it to yourself to limit the amount of stress you feel. The best stress-busting tactics for the workplace include taking five-minute daydreaming breaks every few hours, getting out for a walk at lunchtime and learning to delegate the maddening little details to subordinates. Be aware of your body's response to stress, whether it's a tense jaw, a stiff neck or a headache, and catch the tension before you reach the breaking point.

15. Stay cool at home. The fight against stress continues at home. Experts recommend that you find a private 20 minutes somewhere in your day just for you. You can read or just sit quietly, but the goal is to initiate what doctors call *the relaxation response.* This is a measurable body change that includes a slowing of metabolism, heart rate, rate of breathing *and* blood pressure. The relaxation response dilutes anger, anxiety and depression, says Herbert Benson, M.D., associate professor of medicine at Harvard Medical School.

16. Cut back on salt. If you have high blood pressure, probably the most important thing you can do for the problem is to cut back on salt. "There's no question in my mind that sodium is the major culprit in high blood pressure," says Norman Kaplan, M.D., head of the Hypertension Division at the University of Texas Health Science Center.

An analysis of more than 70 studies concluded that if everyone cut back on daily salt intake by three grams (about 1½ teaspoons), the incidence of stroke would be slashed by 26 percent and one kind of heart disease by 15 percent. Put another way, not salting our food could save an estimated 180,000 American lives each year.

—Greg Gutfeld

Bet against Cancer

Cancer is not inevitable. These do's and don'ts from America's top 200 cancer experts could lower your risk considerably.

If you read the newspapers enough, you might get the impression that just about everything on the planet causes cancer. Hardly a week goes by when there isn't some new front-page scare. In the past few years, everything from apples to water has been implicated as a potential cause of cancer.

This barrage of dire warnings may at times have left you feeling a bit glum. If even fresh fruit and tap water cause cancer, there must be no way to avoid it. And if it's going to get you anyway, why think about it?

Men's Health felt that a little perspective was needed. Cancer strikes only about one in three people. Clearly, it's neither inevitable nor unavoidable for most of us. But because many of the cancer hazards talked about in the media are significantly less worrisome than others, it has become increasingly difficult to get our anticancer priorities straight.

For example, which is more important, checking the radon level in your basement or eating a high-fiber breakfast cereal? Losing weight or avoiding food additives? Going for cancer screenings every year or keeping a positive mental attitude? Knowing these things, it would be possible to develop a rational anticancer plan for yourself.

We felt that the right place to go to get that perspective was to the doctors and scientists on the front lines of cancer research and treatment. We asked Medical Consensus Surveys, a research arm of Rodale Press, to poll 200 experts at the 44 National Cancer Institutes–designated cancer centers in the United States. These physicians and researchers treat large numbers of patients, conduct full-scale tests of new cancer treatments and have access to the most up-to-date information available anywhere.

We asked these specialists to prioritize risk-reducing actions by checking one of five categories: Extremely Important, Very Important, Important, Not Important (But May Help) or Probably Worthless. Their responses were analyzed to reveal a priority list of actions you can take right now to lower your risk of cancer (see "The Top 15 Anticancer Measures" on page 175).

One extremely significant point that emerged from the survey: Half of our experts agreed that 50 to 70 percent of all cancers could be prevented if everybody followed the top-priority changes in lifestyle and diet outlined below.

Kick the Nicotine Habit

As we expected, tobacco use leads the list of risks: Nearly all of our 200 experts say it's extremely important to avoid smoking or chewing tobacco. "If all the smokers in this country quit tomorrow, 30 percent of all cancer deaths could be prevented," says Edward Trapido, Sc.D., an epidemiologist at the University of Miami School of Medicine.

That's not just deaths from lung cancer, either. Smoking causes cancers of the mouth, larynx and esophagus, and in body parts that don't have direct contact with smoke, notably the pancreas and the bladder.

THE TOP 15 ANTICANCER MEASURES

Here's how our experts rated specific actions that can help lower your cancer risk. One action, "Avoid industrial/agricultural toxins" scored high enough (69 percent) to be in fifth place, but it is not included in the top 15. These substances are associated with cancer risks, but exposure to them is confined to workers in certain industries rather than the general population.

Rank	Action
1	Don't smoke or chew tobacco
2	Get regular cancer screening tests
3	Perform testicular self-exams
4	Limit exposure to sunlight
5	Avoid high alcohol intake
6	Avoid "passive smoking"
7	Reduce overall dietary fat
8	Eat more food fiber
9	Eat more fruits and vegetables
10	Eat more whole-grain, high-fiber cereals
11	Maintain normal weight
12	Avoid household toxins
13	Get regular exercise
14	Limit exposure to nitrites
15	Eat more cruciferous vegetables

Tobacco has been a highly publicized risk for nearly 30 years, but the warnings have all been aimed at the smoker. Within the past 10 years, passive smoking—exposure to tobacco smoke from others—has surfaced as a major concern. Over half of our respondents feel that avoiding passive smoking is either very or extremely important.

"The latest information I've read says that a nonsmoker's cancer risk increases 50 percent if he lives with a smoker," says William Shingleton, M.D., retired director of the cancer center at Duke University Medical School. Working eight hours a day in a smoky environment can also raise your risk.

Cut Down on Alcohol

Nearly half the doctors rated avoiding high alcohol intake as very or extremely important. Alcohol in moderation seems to be a negligible risk. But the heavier drinker—14 or more drinks a week—has a greatly increased risk of cancers of the mouth, throat and liver. That's bad enough on its own, but it's a double whammy to the heavy drinker who also smokes, an all-too-common combination.

Avoid Too Much Sun

Essentially all of the more than 500,000 cases of nonmelanoma skin cancer each year are caused by too much sun, says Paul F. Engstrom, M.D., of the Fox Chase Cancer Center in Philadelphia. "The good news is that nonmelanomas are highly treatable, so considerably fewer cancer deaths are attributable to sun exposure."

The bad news: Recent evidence links excessive sun exposure to those rarer-but-deadly melanomas. That's part of the reason that more than two-thirds of our respondents consider sunlight a very to extremely important risk factor.

Get Screened

Regular cancer screening tests and self-exams are methods of early detection rather than cancer prevention. We included them in the survey because early detection leads to a better chance of a cure—preventing deaths rather than the cancer itself. Our respondents agreed. Getting regular checkups and doing self-exams garnered second and third places (after quitting smoking) on the "Top 15" list of cancer-preventing priorities.

The most important do-it-yourself tests for men are testicular self-exams. (After a warm bath or shower, gently roll each testicle between your thumb and fingers, feeling for any hard lumps or irregularities.) Testicular cancer is the leading form among young men, and if detected early it's better than 90 percent curable. It's also smart to keep an eye out for suspected skin cancers. And for men over 40, one of the most important physician-performed screenings is the colorectal cancer test. You can also get screening tests for prostate, skin, thyroid, mouth and lymph cancers.

Keep Weight Down and Exercise Up

As recently as ten years ago, doctors would have dismissed being overweight as a cancer factor. But since then, studies have linked obesity (defined by the American Cancer Society as being 40 percent or more overweight) with increased risk of colon, prostate and gallbladder cancers.

Exercise is crucial in controlling obesity, and our experts rate regular exercise to be of only slightly less importance than maintaining normal weight. It's difficult to establish a *direct* link between exercise and cancer prevention, but some evidence exists, for example, that people with desk jobs and sedentary lives are at higher risk of colorectal cancer. "Exercise may help reduce that risk," says Peter Greenwald, M.D., of the National Cancer Institute headquarters in Bethesda, Maryland.

Think Positively

The notion that mind and body are interrelated is just coming into acceptance by the medical community. Among the doctors in our survey, 54 percent rated having a positive mental attitude as important, very important or extremely important. Only 22 percent labeled it probably worthless. A few years ago, those percentages would easily have been reversed. Recent studies show that stress-reducing techniques can cause measurable changes in the immune system. Whether these changes can help prevent cancer is still speculative at this point. "It's hard to prove scientifically that a positive outlook can help prevent cancer. But many people—doctors, too—have a feeling that people with a positive attitude may smoke less and have better eating habits," says Dr. Greenwald.

Consider Your Environment

Environmental factors scored surprisingly low in importance on our survey. While they are still considered risks, most of our experts think that most are not serious causes of concern.

Electromagnetic fields. About a third of our experts think it's ridiculous to worry about electromagnetic fields from high-tension wires, electric blankets, computer screens and so on. In fact, the magnetic-field category was the second-lowest risk on the entire list. "It's a very, very, very rare cause of cancer compared with smoking and sun exposure. But people tend to overestimate the risk of outside factors they can't control," Dr. Engstrom explains.

Radon. This one is a little more controversial. The Environmental Protection Agency maintains that radon is the second most important cause of lung cancer, right after smoking. The EPA's warning is based primarily on studies of miners exposed to radon miles underground. Can we accurately relate those findings to the risk aboveground?

"I don't believe there's a shred of epidemiological data to relate household radon exposure to cancer—nothing that links cancer clusters and high-radon areas," states J. John Cohen, M.D., Ph.D., of the University of Colorado Medical School. Yet probably because the American Cancer Society backs radon as a potential risk factor, 47 percent of our doctors still say it's important to check the radon level in your home. The rest seem to be on the fence: Over 26 percent say it isn't important but it may help. Very few of the experts picked the extreme responses.

Toxins. Industrial and agricultural toxins scored high as risk factors. There is solid research linking certain industrial agents (such as nickel, chromate, asbestos and vinyl chloride) to increased cancer risks in workers. Farm pesticides may also pose hazards to farmers. But the risks are limited since only a relatively small part of the population works with carcinogenic chemicals on a daily basis.

Twenty years ago, you'd be hard-pressed to find a doctor who'd say that diet had anything to do with preventing cancer. Things have changed dramatically, and our survey shows it. Most of our experts rated dietary habits important, very important or extremely important.

"Dietary factors probably account for up to 35 percent of all cancers. That's according to a landmark National Cancer Institute–sponsored report," Dr. Trapido states. And this figure is higher than the figure for smoking. (Not a big surprise since everybody eats and only a minority still smoke.)

Chemicals in your food. There are a number of items in our survey that can be termed "dietary chemical hazards." Like the environmental risk factors above, these chemicals have reputations that are far worse than their scores on this survey.

Nitrites, which are used to cure bacon, hot dogs and other meats, received the most concern from our experts. Nitrites have indeed been associated with increased cancer risks.

Washing fruits and vegetables to remove chemical residues may be a good health practice, but it counts as only a moderate risk reducer.

Concern with food additives scored toward the bottom of the list in importance. As with other chemicals, frequency of exposure is the key to determining risk. Eating fresh fruits and vegetables and avoiding high-fat prepared foods limits contact with preservatives.

Our experts considered irradiated foods as virtually a nonexistent risk. The irradiation is done to kill bacteria and extend shelf life. "It does not make food radioactive, and there is no known cancer risk," reports L. M. Glode, M.D., of the University of Colorado Cancer Center.

The bottom lines: If you still smoke, give it up; don't be shy about asking your doctor for a cancer screening; stay out of the noon-day sun; consume less alcohol and fat and more fruits, vegetables and other fiber-rich foods; and, finally, stop worrying about all that other cancer stuff you read about in the newspapers.

—Steven Lally

No More Back Pain

You can turn a bad back into a good back. Just 15 minutes a day can give you a lifetime of freedom from back pain.

Back experts agree that one of the best ways to avoid back pain is to exercise: If you keep your body flexible, strong and well conditioned, they say, you're far less likely to get a backache.

Still, simply being active isn't enough, since back pain hits active men, too. (Sports greats Joe Montana, Larry Bird, Don Mattingly, Jack Nicklaus and Mario Lemieux all have bum backs.)

If you're among the 53 percent of men who have been laid low by back pain, you know what a downright frustrating and debilitating experience it can be. You're in agony, you can't work, you can't play, you can't walk, you can't get in and out of bed on your own, let alone make love while you're there. Back pain makes weak men out of strong ones.

WHO'LL STOP THE PAIN?

Who is most likely to provide relief from back pain? An orthopedist? A neurologist? How about a neurosurgeon? The answer—at least in one survey of 492 back-pain sufferers—is none of the above.

Practitioner	Moderate to Dramatic Long-Term Relief (%)	Temporary Relief (%)
Yoga instructors	96	4
Physiatrists	86	0
Physical therapists	65	0
Acupuncturists	36	32
Chiropractors	28	28
Osteopathic physicians	28	15
Neurosurgeons	26	8
Orthopedists	23	9
Family practitioners	20	14
Massage therapists	10	63
Neurologists	4	4

But you don't have to take back pain lying down. The experts are right about the importance of exercise, but it's important to get the right kind. If your fitness regimen consists of playing tennis a couple times a week, hefting weights solely to build killer biceps and riding your bike on weekends, you qualify as active, but you aren't doing much that will help build a stronger back. To do that, you have to target your back for its own exercise program.

Despite all the scary talk you hear about blown disks and degenerating joints, the vast majority of painful back episodes are caused by muscle strain, which, among active men, usually comes from two things, says Mitch Bogdanffy, an exercise physiologist at the Texas Back Institute (TBI).

The first is demanding more of back muscles than they can handle: lifting heavy objects improperly (the familiar advice to lift with the legs, keeping the back straight and objects close to the body, is ignored with astonishing regularity) or going overboard on leisure activities such as sports and gardening.

Take It Easy at First

You're particularly at risk of throwing out your back with racket sports, golf, bowling, football, canoeing, baseball, basketball or anything requiring lots of arching, twisting and sudden starts and stops. To minimize back strain from these sports, it's best to take it easy at the start of the season or when first learning, always easing muscles in and out of activity with warm-ups, cool-downs and stretches.

A second cause of strain is weak muscles, especially in the abdomen. Strong abdominal muscles help to stabilize the lower back, the spine's most vulnerable point. Weak ones allow an exaggerated curve in the lower back, a posture that crimps muscles, nerves and disks.

One study found back-pain sufferers to have just as much back-muscle endurance as healthier people, but weaker stomach muscles. You don't have to be doing anything particularly strenuous to throw out your back if the abdominal muscles are soft—many men report being flattened by pain while bending over to tie a shoelace or pat the dog, or reaching around to grab a briefcase off the car seat. These actions by themselves don't cause the backache; they're just the last straw.

"A weak belly strains the muscles that run along the lower spine," explains physical therapist and fitness author Carol Greenburg. "They are always being pulled, they are always resisting, and they simply get exhausted from the effort. Simple exhaustion can throw a muscle into spasm, a contraction that feels like a knot, hurts like the devil and won't let go for days."

If your problem is weak abdominals (which it probably is if you're not currently doing anything specific to strengthen them), boosting the muscles with exercise is the best thing you can do to protect your back.

The YMCA Healthy Back Program, a respected exercise regimen that dates back to the 1940s, devotes its strengthening exercises almost exclusively to the abdominals. In an evaluation of 233 patients who took part in the program, 82 percent found that their usual back pain either stopped or decreased significantly. Only 2.5 percent of the participants showed little or no improvement.

Specifically, here's how building strong stomach muscles can help bolster your back.

It stabilizes the spine. "The abdominal muscles and the low back muscles together form a column of muscles that must be strong all around," says Wayne Westcott, Ph.D., YMCA national strength-training consultant. When strong and balanced, these trunk muscles ease the spine's weight-carrying and structural burden. "But if one side is weak, it may put excess stress on the spine and the nerves and tissue that surround it," Dr. Westcott says.

It cuts flab. A potbelly can make spinal instability worse. "For Americans, the abdomen is exercised very little, and it's where body fat tends to migrate," says Dr. Westcott. It's a double whammy, like sending extra traffic to a congested bridge with weak supports. Something's got to give—in this case, your spine. Coupling a low-fat diet with a full exercise program that emphasizes abdominals may be as close as you can get to natural liposuction for the gut.

It eases everyday movements. A strong abdomen helps the body cope with everyday resistive activities, whether moving furniture or climbing stairs, lugging a heavy suitcase or catching a ball. "If those abdominal muscles are weak, you'll overcompensate with your back," says TBI physical therapist Paula Gilbert. "This can lead to a back sprain over and over again. You need to have these stomach and back muscles synergized—working together—or your back will not respond well after injury."

Get Strong All Over

Zeroing in on your stomach muscles makes almost no sense, however, if you neglect everything else. At the Texas Back Institute, specialists emphasize the importance of cardiovascular fitness for decreasing back pain and injury, and recommend aerobic exercise—walking, swimming, water exercises, stationary cycling—for any back-building program.

"Cardiovascular exercise lubricates the joints and stretches muscles so they're less prone to strain and tearing," says Stephen Hochschuler, M.D., surgeon and TBI cofounder. Research backs this up: A study of 1,652 firefighters found that the most cardiovascularly fit of them had ten times fewer debilitating back injuries than the least fit.

Exercise also promotes the efficient transport of oxygen to muscles, which helps healing, and boosts daily production of your body's self-made painkillers, endorphins and enkephalins.

To strengthen specific muscles that support the spine and help the back do its job, you also need to include the abdominals, the oblique muscles (running from the back of the spine to the front of the abdomen), the extensor muscles of the lower back and the leg muscles that share lifting duty.

The following routine hits them all, but especially works those abdominals. You can do the complete workout at home in less than 15 minutes.

First, some pointers:

• To get the most back-boosting benefits, do the exercises three times a week or more.

• Exercise with slow, controlled movements: Speed adds momentum, momentum carries you, and the muscles end up doing less work.

• Avoid full sit-ups, which use only about 30 percent of the abdominal muscles, leaving the hip flexors to do most of the work. If you rise only slightly, your abdominals will do 90 percent of the work.

• When you're performing these exercises, put something between you and the ground. A body-length mat, available at just about any sporting goods store, cushions your back much better than a cold, hard floor.

• People with back pain can usually do light exercises. But see a doctor first if no position gives you relief, if your pain has lasted more than two weeks, if it radiates down your leg to your knee or foot or if simple movement makes the pain worse.

Now, your routine:

Pelvic tilt. This exercise primarily strengthens abdominal muscles, but it also builds muscles in the lower back that keep it properly aligned with the pelvis.

Lie on your back, with your knees raised and your arms extended to the side. Press your lower back against the floor by tightening the abdominal muscles and squeezing the buttocks. Hold for ten seconds. Repeat five to ten times.

Partial curl. This targets the rectus abdominis muscles at the front of the body.

Lie on your back with your knees bent. Extend your hands straight out between your thighs. Slowly curl your upper torso until your shoulder blades leave the floor, exhaling while rising. Hold for ten seconds. Do 5 reps the first week, then increase by 5 a week until you can do 15.

Advanced curl. Move on to this exercise when you can easily do 20 partial curls.

Lie on your back with your knees bent and your fingers lightly touching your ears. Slowly curl your upper torso until your shoulders leave the floor, exhaling. Hold for ten seconds. Start with 5 reps, increasing by fives as they get easy.

Twist curl. This works the obliques, or side abdominal muscles.

Lie on your back with your knees bent. Fold your arms across your chest. Slowly curl your right shoulder off the floor toward the left knee until your left shoulder leaves the floor. Hold for ten seconds, breathing deeply. Repeat, but with your left shoulder toward your right knee. Do three of each.

Spinal extension. This strengthens the lumbar extensor muscles of the lower back.

Lie face down on your stomach with your elbows bent and your fingers lightly touching your ears. Lift your upper body off the floor, exhaling. Hold for ten seconds. Do 5 reps to start, then add two a week until you can do 15 to 20.

Advanced spinal extension. Start this exercise when you can do 15 to 20 spinal extensions.

Use the same position as in the spinal extension, but with your arms extended straight out in front of you. Do 5 reps to start, increasing by twos as they become easy.

Leg extension. This strengthens the quadriceps.

Sit on a surface that allows your legs to dangle straight down from the knee without touching the ground. Wearing ankle weights, straighten one leg in a slow, controlled motion. Repeat with the other leg. The weight should be heavy enough to slightly fatigue muscles after 12 reps. Increase to 15 reps after the first week. After two weeks at 15 reps, boost the weight by five pounds.

—Greg Gutfeld

Farewell to Knee Pain

Treat your knees right, and they'll carry you the distance. Here's how to get a leg up on the most common of problems.

It's not really fair the way knee injuries occur. Take the case of Gerry, an engineer in his forties, whose knee started acting up after a minor ski accident. (A less experienced skier rammed him from behind—while he was getting off the lift, no less.) Gerry's no sofa pilot. He keeps in shape, and he's devoted to a number of outdoor sports. His doctor had him in a leg immobilizer for a while, then put him on a regimen of leg-strengthening exercises. Pretty soon—too soon—Gerry was back to one of his favorite sports: speedwalking. His rehab, however, had built up only some of the muscles in his injured leg, and that caused an imbalance. The result was a classic case of runner's knee.

Whether we're young, old or middle-aged, the knee is our most vulnerable joint. It's also a repeat offender: Once you've seriously injured a knee, your odds of reinjuring it are astronomical. But you can beat those odds if you practice a little prevention and get prompt medical attention at the first sign of trouble.

Why is the knee such a sore spot? Partly because it's not one of nature's best engineering jobs. "The knee is essentially a ball sitting on a flat surface, held in place by four rubber bands," says James Fox, M.D., an orthopedic surgeon and author of the book *Save Your Knees*. "It's a perfectly good joint—for an animal that lived millions of years ago and walked on all fours."

Those of us who live today and walk on two legs tend to put a lot of stress and strain on our knees. We gain weight. We try to lose it by jogging, skiing, playing football and basketball. We get a little pain, but we write it off to being "out of shape." Even worse, we try to work through the discomfort. The words of Little League and junior-varsity coaches from our past egg us on: "Whatsa matter *(your name here)*? Gonna let a little *pain* slow you down? My grandmother can move faster than that, and she uses a walker!"

But "no pain, no gain" is the *wrong* philosophy, especially when

TWIN PEAKS: PUMPING UP YOUR KNEES

The best way to prevent a knee injury is to keep the muscles that operate the knees in peak condition. That's what these exercises are designed to do. Just be sure to get your doctor's okay first, as some of these exercises could aggravate preexisting injuries, especially if done too soon or with too much weight.

You can do most of these exercises on the kind of weight machines found at a gym, or you can buy ankle weights for home use. Two inexpensive alternatives: penny rolls (about three to a pound) and lead fishing sinkers. Put them in a sock, knot the end securely, and drape the sock over your ankle. When you work up to more weight, you can put your pennies in a runner's fanny pack and hang the strap over your ankle.

If any of these exercises hurt, stop immediately. Try less weight or no weight. You want to feel muscle burn, but pain anywhere in the joint is a signal to back off.

1. Straight-leg raise. Lie on your back on a firm surface. Bend one leg at the knee, keeping the foot flat on the floor. Lock the knee of the other leg in an extended position and lift from the hip. Raise your foot no more than 6 or 8 inches and hold for about 6 seconds. Then drop your leg and rest for 6

dealing with knees. Pain in the joint itself indicates a problem that can only get worse if not treated. Fortunately, in nine out of ten cases, knee problems can be treated rather conservatively, with immediate rest and subsequent physical therapy. In cases where a knee injury does require surgery, a thin, tubelike instrument called an arthroscope makes it possible to do complex repairs through a few small holes in the skin, greatly reducing recovery time.

Gerry took his knee to Elliott B. Hershman, M.D., an orthopedic surgeon at the Nicholas Institute of Sports Medicine at Lenox Hill Hospital in New York City. Dr. Hershman prescribed hip-abductor exercises to strengthen the quadriceps. "By bending at the hip instead of the knee, Gerry worked the muscles without aggravating the injured seconds. Do ten repetitions of this exercise with your right leg, then ten with your left leg.

You may want to start without weights. Gradually add weight as you gain strength—up to about 5 pounds maximum. Then, rather than adding weight, see if you can hold your leg up for 10 seconds instead of 6 without shaking. You can eventually build up to three sets of ten repetitions.

2. Seated quadriceps extensions. Sit in a chair with your legs bent at the knee and hanging down. With a comfortable amount of ankle weight, raise your legs two-thirds of the way and hold for six seconds, then rest. Repeat ten times. Don't extend your legs straight out, because the extra stress will do more harm than good. Gym version: This exercise can be duplicated at the gym on a thigh-and-knee weight machine.

3. Hamstring strengthener. Stand facing a wall, with your hands braced against it for stability. With your ankle weight secured, lift your foot and slowly bring your shin to a 90-degree angle with the floor. Hold for 6 seconds, then slowly lower your foot. Do ten repetitions with each foot. This exercise can be duplicated on a thigh-and-knee weight machine. The only difference is that you lie on your stomach, pulling the weight until your feet are pointing straight up.

joint," Dr. Hershman explains. How does Gerry feel now? "Great! A year after the injury I was back on the slopes," he says. And for an active man, that is the true test of any cure.

Get a Leg Up on the Problem

The kneecap, or patella, is the focus of the most common kind of knee pain: chondromalacia patella. It's often called runner's knee, but it strikes nonrunners as well—as Gerry could tell you.

Runner's knee can feel like a generalized, dull ache in the front of the knee or a very specific, sharp pain of the inner surface of the kneecap. The pain is caused by damage to the cartilage behind the kneecap. "The first stage is a softening of the cartilage, but eventually it gets chewed up," says Lyle L. Micheli, M.D., president of the American College of Sports Medicine and associate professor of orthopedics at Harvard University. "It's the result of excess or uneven pressure on the kneecap during activity."

If you have runner's knee, it's of primary importance to stop aggravating the injury. "The first thing I get my patients to do is cut back to a comfortable level of activity," says James G. Garrick, M.D., an orthopedic surgeon and director of the Center for Sports Medicine at St. Francis Memorial Hospital in San Francisco.

When the knee stops hurting, that's half the battle. The other half is for your doctor to figure out exactly how the knee got hurt. Three frequently interrelated problems cause runner's knee.

1. Overtraining or starting a new workout: Trying to do too much too soon can wreak havoc on more than your knees.

2. Hidden weaknesses: Sometimes one of the four muscles that make up the quadriceps isn't pulling its own weight. Often this is the vastus medialis, which keeps the kneecap on the right track as it moves up and down. It's also possible for the hamstrings (rear thigh muscles) and calf muscles to be too tight in relation to the quadriceps.

3. Structural flaws: Barely noticeable misalignments of the leg and foot cause the kneecap not to move properly in its groove. These can be problems you're born with, like being knock-kneed or pigeon-toed, or they can be brought on by external factors, such as too much running on an uneven surface.

While strengthening—usually starting with gentle-on-the-joints isometric exercises and graduating to light weight lifting—can correct training errors and muscle imbalances, it can't help all cases of misalignment. Sometimes prescription orthotic insoles are required.

More aggressive tactics include putting the patient on crutches for a few weeks and, rarely, giving injections of anti-inflammatory drugs. Surgery is a last resort.

One procedure for misalignment problems involves partially severing some of the tendons that attach to the outer edge of the kneecap. This allows the quadriceps to pull the kneecap inward and back into line. The other surgical option is to smooth down the cartilage surfaces on the front of the thigh bone and behind the kneecap through arthroscopic surgery.

The next most common knee injury is a cartilage tear, although perhaps that's a misleading term. "It's not surface cartilage that tears, but two movable cartilage shock absorbers in the knee called menisci," explains Robert Bielen, M.D., a sports medicine specialist and clinical assistant professor at the University of California, Irvine.

A tear is often caused by a specific accident. Sam, a hotel manager in his fifties, had just crossed the finish line of a Central Park road race when another runner rammed into him. "He was showing off for the TV cameras. I landed on my knees and heard a pop. The medics cleaned out the scrapes and told me I'd be fine. But over the next few months, I noticed the knee bothered me whenever I ran," he remembers.

Symptoms of a meniscal tear are sharp pain at the joint line when you move and slipping or locking of the joint. Tears generally don't heal on their own—especially tears toward the meniscus center, where blood supply is poor. "But there's good evidence that a tear on the edge of the meniscus will heal, especially if it's stitched up," says Dr. Micheli. When the tear is in the middle of the meniscus, surgeons just try to smooth out the rough spots. The most common way is to shave down the ragged edges of the tear with tiny instruments manipulated through an arthroscope. Another approach is to zap the edges of the tear with a laser, a relatively uncommon but effective procedure.

Sam, who, like Gerry, was a patient of Dr. Hershman, was advised to have surgery, since the tear was on the edge of the meniscus. "It was a flap tear that wouldn't compromise the shock-absorbing qualities of the meniscus, so I removed the torn flap," Dr. Hershman explains. Sam is back to running every day: "A year later, and I can't even find the scars!"

Tears That Bring Tears

Torn ligaments are also responsible for knee pain. Of the four ligaments that stabilize the knee, the one most likely to stretch or snap is the anterior cruciate ligament, or ACL. That's because the ACL stabilizes the knee from front to back—the direction in which you're most likely to overstress it. The ACL keeps the tibia (shin bone) from sliding forward and out from under the femur.

Ligaments can stretch about 6 percent of their length. After that, they snap. "You can have a partial tear of the ACL," says Dr. Micheli, "but most are clean breaks." This injury usually occurs during sudden stops and twists in football or soccer or when jumping and landing in basketball or volleyball. If you pull one of these moves and hear a loud pop, chances are you've snapped the ACL. Swelling follows.

"I didn't hear a pop, but I had only a partial tear of the ligament—at first," says Andrew, a lawyer in his late twenties. He was playing a friendly game of basketball when he twisted the wrong way during an attempted hot-shot move. "I fell face down in horrible pain. It was so bad I had difficulty breathing," he recalls. "My first reaction was to try to walk it off, but it quickly became apparent I needed to go to a doctor."

Most ACL tears are diagnosed by a physical exam and the patient's description of what happened. Two high-tech methods can be used to confirm the diagnosis: arthroscopic examination and magnetic resonance imaging (MRI). (Ligaments don't show up clearly on x-rays.) Andrew underwent an MRI and was told his ligament was severed. But then a closer look through an arthroscope showed that he actually had 30 percent of the ligament left intact. If the blood flow to the ACL wasn't disrupted, there would be a chance of saving it.

Surgery isn't required in every instance of an ACL tear or break, but not fixing the damage will limit a person's mobility somewhat. Simple exercises to strengthen the muscles around the knee can give adequate stability for most everyday activities. "The first doctor I went to told me to learn to love biking and golfing," says Andrew. You can also walk, run and swim with a severed ACL. But climbing, carrying heavy objects or walking on uneven ground is difficult.

Andrew eventually had to undergo ligament-replacement surgery when his ACL deteriorated because of poor blood flow. There are three types of replacement ligaments, listed here in order of preference:

• A transplant from the patient's own body, using part of either a leg tendon or hamstring

• A part-natural, part-synthetic transplant called a stent, in which a tiny piece of polypropylene rope strengthens a replacement tendon

• A completely artificial tendon made of Gore-Tex (yes, it's the same thing they make raincoats from).

Andrew's doctor, Ralph A. Gambardella, M.D., an orthopedic surgeon at the Kerlan-Jobe Orthopedic Clinic in Inglewood, California, chose to transplant a piece of Andrew's own patellar tendon, which runs from the kneecap to the shin. In general, the success rate with ligament-replacement surgery is 90 percent or better, but the road to full recovery is long and requires sticking to a strict physical-therapy regimen.

"My knee will never be exactly the same, but I've come a lot farther after a few months of rehab than I ever expected," Andrew says. "After the injury, I swore I'd never set foot on a basketball court again. Now, Dr. Gambardella actually encourages me to play slow-motion one-on-one as part of my therapy. My hook-shot days might not be over just yet."

—Steven Lally

The Wonder Drug in Your Medicine Cabinet

Take a look at aspirin's newly discovered benefits. You may be in for a few pleasant surprises.

Perhaps it's time to stop thinking of aspirin as that 100-tablets-for-$1.99 pain reliever you take when you have a mild headache. Although it's been a medicine-cabinet staple for more than 100 years, researchers have been taking a new look at it, and some of their conclusions are startling. In fact, when you look at all the therapeutic claims made lately for aspirin, you might wonder what ills it *won't* prevent—sometimes even with small doses.

Men's Health sent its research staff out to explore the latest aspirin studies. The researchers turned up the following list of the drug's newly discovered benefits.

Reduces Risk of Heart Attack

Aspirin's role in preventing heart attacks is probably its strongest credential. There now seems little question that an aspirin tablet every other day can help prevent first heart attacks and can be helpful to those who've had one already.

How does it work? First, we know that aspirin's main biological effect is to limit the production of substances called prostaglandins. And we know that one of the duties of prostaglandins is to promote blood clotting. So regular doses of aspirin help keep blood from clumping together, which reduces the likelihood that an artery will plug up and cause a heart attack.

In the Physicians' Health Study, a long-term study of over 22,000 healthy male doctors, those who took a standard 325-milligram aspirin tablet every other day had 44 percent fewer heart attacks than those who didn't. The researchers were so impressed by the results they stopped the trial in midcourse and put all the doctors on aspirin.

Reduces Risk of Stroke

While nearly all research has shown that aspirin reduces the risk of heart disease, its effect on stroke is much more controversial. Of ten major studies conducted between 1977 and 1988, six have shown a reduction in stroke risk for those taking aspirin, while four have shown no effect. So the results are less than conclusive.

When these studies are divided into categories, however, some patterns emerge. First, aspirin has been shown in most trials to reduce the chance of recurrence in those who've already *had* a stroke. And second, it seems to help those who have other circulatory problems, such as irregular heart rhythm, chest pains and heart disease. In one study, patients with a rhythm problem called atrial fibrillation had 50 to 80 percent fewer strokes when given aspirin.

Reduces Risk of Colon Cancer

An American team reported in the *Journal of the National Cancer Institute* that when they compared 1,326 colorectal cancer patients with 4,891 cancer-free patients, those without tumors were much more likely to be regular aspirin users. In fact, the aspirin users turned out to have one-half the risk of developing this disease.

Reduces Risk of Cataracts

The risk of getting cataracts is related to blood glucose levels, and there's some evidence that aspirin reduces the rate at which the body uses glucose. So British researchers tried administering aspirin and the aspirin-like medication ibuprofen to 300 patients. They found that the users of both drugs were half as likely to develop cataracts.

Boosts the Immune System

Aspirin has been found to increase the production of three important immune system chemicals: interleukin-2, interferon-gamma and interferon-alpha.

While researching this effect, scientists also tested aspirin's potential for warding off a cold. Although the subjects enjoyed no added protection from that common ailment, they did produce less mucus when they caught a cold.

Protects against Gallstones

Scientists in the United States and Britain decided to see how aspirin would affect people with known gallstone risk factors such as high-calcium or reduced-calorie diets. Reporting in *Lancet* on 75 of the at-risk people they surveyed, the British researchers found that the 12 regular aspirin users developed no gallstones, while 20 of the 63 nonusers did. In the *New England Journal of Medicine,* U.S. scientists reported that of 68 adults on weight-loss diets, aspirin users developed fewer gallstones than those given a placebo.

Reduces Frequency of Migraine Headaches

Aspirin is not a remedy for a full-blown migraine attack, but taking it on a regular basis seems to reduce the *frequency* of the attacks. In the Physicians' Health Study, doctors taking aspirin every other day reported 20 percent fewer migraine attacks than those who got placebos. This finding is supported by a similar British study that showed regular doses of aspirin led to a 29 percent reduction in migraines.

Relieves Hay Fever Symptoms

According to a report in the *Annals of Allergy,* aspirin is as effective as some antihistamines in treating pollen allergies. One 41-year-old allergy sufferer enjoyed relief from symptoms for up to eight hours after taking aspirin.

May Become a Flu Cure

According to a letter in the *New England Journal of Medicine,* aspirin in very high doses can completely halt the activity of influenza virus. The dosage required is far too high to be given orally to humans, but researchers speculate that an aerosol form sprayed into the nose might someday be effective in controlling flu in the respiratory system.

Aspirin is so inexpensive and readily available that it's easy to forget it really is a drug. In fact, it's so potent, many researchers think that if aspirin were discovered or invented today, the Food and Drug Admini-stration would restrict its availability to prescriptions. The main reason you can buy it freely is that it has been around so long.

WHY NOT ONCE A DAY?

In a British study of over 5,000 doctors, a daily dose of aspirin did not significantly protect the doctors from heart attack, but an aspirin *every other day* did. Yes, it would be a lot simpler to take an aspirin every day—or even half an aspirin. Unfortunately, that simply doesn't work.

One explanation has to do with the specific prostaglandins that aspirin affects. For example, aspirin suppresses thromboxane, a blood thickener. Unfortunately, it also suppresses prostacyclin, a prostaglandin that inhibits blood clot formation.

It seems that when you take a dose every other day, blood-thinning prostacyclin has time to return to normal, while blood-thickening thromboxane stays suppressed, producing a net gain in blood-thinning potential.

Another reason to stick to an every-other-day dose has to do with immune system enhancement. When researchers gave their subjects aspirin every day, their immune systems were boosted at first but then ebbed back to normal levels. When the people got aspirin on alternate days, however, immune levels remained at a much higher level.

Aspirin is not without its side effects when used in large doses. It can slow blood clotting, produce ulcers and cause tinnitus, an annoying ringing in the ears.

It would be wise to talk to your doctor before beginning a regular course of aspirin. Even if he says okay, don't overdo it. The optimum dose for cardiac benefits seems to be one regular strength (325-milligram) tablet every other day. When you take it in higher doses or more frequently, not only do the side effects increase but some of the benefits may disappear as well (see "Why Not Once a Day?" on the opposite page).

That being said, taking aspirin may well be the cheapest, most effective preventive there is—other than regular exercise and eating less fat—for a variety of illnesses.

—Dave Schoonmaker

Dangerous Pleasures

When is too much really too much? Here's a party pooper's guide to the dangers lurking in life's little pleasures.

There really *can* be too much of a good thing. Not just too much money, which would surely spoil us (or so our bosses keep pointing out), but too much of normal, everyday pleasures like exercise, sleep, even water. How much is too much? In most cases *a lot,* but for those people who just never know when to stop, *Men's Health* has prepared this guide.

Alcohol

Within 60 minutes of downing three or more alcoholic drinks, glasses of wine or bottles of beer, your blood alcohol level can top 0.10. That's enough to get you busted for driving while intoxicated in most states. Twenty-five drinks in an hour can kill you, a fact that has been tragically verified at college fraternity parties over the years. The overdose of alcohol shuts down your central nervous system to the point where your brain stops sending out signals reminding you to breathe.

Caffeine

Caffeine is strong stuff. The amount in five or six cups of coffee—or 12 cans of cola—can make you anxious, restless, jittery. Forty cups can create symptoms that mimic severe mental illness or even a heart attack.

Carrots

Eating more than five to six carrots per day for several months can turn your skin orange. The harmless discoloration is caused by orange pigment from the beta-carotene in the carrots and disappears once you reduce your intake. Although the problem may not help you make any new friends, it's not dangerous: You'd have to eat about 318,000 carrots to get a toxic dose of beta-carotene.

Credit Cards

Carrying a wallet stuffed with too many credit cards can cause an irritation of the nerve that runs down the buttocks into the thigh, a condition doctors refer to as "creditcarditis."

Fiber

It's hard to overdose on dietary fiber, since you'd tend to start feeling very full before you reached the danger zone. If you could manage to eat six bowls of high-fiber cereal at one sitting, you'd probably wind up with a bad stomachache from all those carbohydrates fermenting in your gut.

Fiber pills used for weight loss are another story. Some doctors have reported cases, albeit rare ones, of blocked esophagi from fiber pills expanding as patients swallowed them.

Heat

Exercising vigorously in 90° heat can raise your body temperature to 103° or higher, causing headaches and difficulty breathing. It's not a good idea to exercise outdoors on very hot days. If you must, drink about a half a glass of water every 10 to 15 minutes while you're working out.

Hot Tubbing

It's risky to drink liquor while you're in a hot tub because alcohol inhibits the body's temperature-regulation system. The hot water could raise your body temperature to a dangerous level and even cause your blood pressure to plunge. Should that happen, you could pass out and drown.

Music

Over time, loud music destroys the tiny hairs in the ear canal that register sound waves. The louder the music, the less time this takes. For example, sitting in front of a wall of amplifiers at a rock concert for two hours is enough to do some permanent damage to your hearing.

Playing Pool

Playing pool for eight hours straight can produce a sharp pain in your cue-pushing shoulder. Apparently the syndrome is caused by the extension and rotation of the shoulder required by the game—an action that can compress veins of the upper chest against the first rib, causing a pain-producing blood clot.

Push-Ups

Doing as few as 20 to 30 push-ups a day on a hard surface may cause "push-up palsy," a numbness of the hand caused by pinching the nerve that runs through the palm. If you do a lot of push-ups, get yourself a padded mat.

Salt

Your body needs a mere 500 milligrams of salt—$\frac{1}{16}$ teaspoon—per day. You can get that in a cup of instant soup or a few handfuls of honey-roasted peanuts. The average American man eats 20 times that amount. When you begin to approach 20 to 30 grams per day (which, incidentally, is what the average Japanese consumes), you get to a level that may put you at risk for high blood pressure, arterial damage and even stroke.

Sex

We're happy to report that you can't have too much sex. Even the party poopers can't find anything wrong with overindulging here. In fact, the chances of dying in the act are so slim as to be nearly nonexistent. In a study of 5,550 men who died suddenly, only 34 of them perished during sex.

Sleep

Sleeping more than ten hours nightly may shorten your life. A study of a million adults found that the mortality rate for long sleepers was 1½ to 2 times greater than the rate for people who slept seven to eight hours. Major causes of death were heart disease, cancer and suicide.

Soda

Six to seven cans of regular *or* diet soda daily can wreak havoc on your teeth. It's not just the sugar but also citric and phosphoric acids, commonly used flavor enhancers, that are to blame. The soda's acidity will, over time, erode tooth enamel.

Spinach

Eating more than three cups of spinach a week may weaken your bones. Researchers found that oxalate, a compound in spinach, blocks absorption of calcium, which in turn may result in weak, fracture-prone bones when you hit your later years.

Telephoning

For those with sensitive skin, eight hours on the telephone can lead to listening-in dermatitis, an irritation of the skin on the cheeks. The constant friction between the phone and the skin combined with perspiration and dirt from hands and the telephone receiver provides a healthy breeding ground for bacteria. The rash is common among telephone salesmen.

Tooth Brushing

Too-vigorous brushing can lacerate the gum tissue and cause bleeding. Repeated rough teeth cleaning will permanently wear away enamel and cause gums to recede. To brush properly, hold your toothbrush with your fingers rather than in your fist. Start by placing the brush just below the gum line. Then brush down on upper teeth; up on lower teeth. Always use a brush labeled "soft."

Vacation

Yes, you can get too much vacation, especially if you're a Type A. Allen Elkin, Ph.D., director of the Stress Management and Counseling Center in New York, tells us that most men begin to crave stimulation as they approach two weeks of a very relaxing vacation. If they don't get it, then the lack of stimulation creates the kind of stress they were often fleeing from in the first place. "You'll develop symptoms of stress—tension, headache, in some it's fatigue. You actually burn out from vacation," says Dr. Elkin.

Vitamin A

A dose of 50,000 international units of vitamin A is toxic to humans. Several early Arctic explorers learned this lesson the hard way when they killed polar bears and ate the livers. Polar bears ingest huge quantities of fish, and *millions* of units of vitamin A are concentrated in their livers. The explorers developed drowsiness, irritability, headache and vomiting. A few days later, their skin began to peel off. The fact that only some lived to tell the tale proves that too much vitamin A can kill.

Water

The typical man at rest needs about 1½ to 2 quarts of water a day (about six to eight glasses). Fifteen to 20 quarts in a day could potentially overwhelm the kidneys' ability to excrete the liquid, resulting in water intoxication. Symptoms include nausea, lightheadedness and even seizures. In severe cases, this can be fatal.

—S. Peter Davidson

199

PART 8

Looking Good

Hair Care 101

If shinier, cleaner, healthier hair is what you're after, read this chapter. Let the experts teach you a thing or two about good-looking locks.

Guys aren't supposed to care about their hair. We know this; you know this; shampoo companies know this. To think about such things would be an admission of vanity. Most men would sooner confess that they voted for Richard Nixon (twice) than acknowledge that they give more than an occasional passing thought to their looks.

So admit nothing. Just read on, out of idle curiosity, as we explain how a *theoretical* head of hair might be made to look consistently shiny, clean and healthy. You don't have to worry about what it means to be learning this stuff, since, if you recall, you never asked.

Cleanliness Is Next to Nothing

We'll start with shine. Shine is directly related to the health and cleanliness of each hair's outer layer, called the cuticle. Seven layers of clear cuticle cells help keep harmful chemicals from penetrating the inner core of the hair and causing damage. The cuticle also holds in moisture needed to keep hair supple. Healthy cuticle cells lie flat, overlapping slightly, like shingles on a roof. When light hits them, it's reflected smoothly, creating shine. Anything that scatters the reflection or dulls the cuticle lessens the gleam.

The cuticle can be damaged by any number of things—sweat, dust, dirt, heat, solar radiation, chlorine and air pollution. When this happens, the cells lift like shingles in a storm, and the roughed-up surfaces don't reflect light in the same direction. The result is dull-looking, and often hopelessly tangled, hair.

The solution can be as simple as choosing the right shampoo. The average has 15 ingredients, formulated to clean hair without drying it out. (Some experts believe that the more ingredients a shampoo contains, the better it is.) The cleansing action of a shampoo is provided by a group of cosmetic ingredients called surfactants, a fancy name for detergents that loosen oil, dirt, dead cells and other debris so that they can be rinsed away easily. By combining the right surfactants with other cosmetic ingredients, a basic cleansing shampoo can be developed for oily, normal or dry hair. (Despite some claims, there's no such thing as a "self-adjusting" shampoo that's right for all types of hair.)

"Start by looking for a reputable brand that states on the label that it's for your hair type," says John Corbett, Ph.D., vice-president of technology at Clairol. "But there's no single surfactant that's the best for everyone with your hair type. So you may have to try a few before you find which works best for you."

You'll also want to look for a shampoo that's pH-balanced (meaning a pH between 5 and 6). A shampoo with a pH below 5 is too acid and won't lather well, and lathering action is essential for removing dirt and dust.

If you swim in pools regularly, you may need to use a shampoo that's formulated to remove chlorine from the hair. There are several brands available, among them UltraSwim, Revitalize and Swimmer.

There's Oil in Them There Hairs

Excessive oiliness is a common problem, particularly among men with blond hair. "The texture of your hair makes a difference. Oil wicks onto fine, straight hair very easily. But wiry hair doesn't seem oily. It has a lot to do with perception," says Thomas Goodman, Jr., M.D., an assistant professor of dermatology at the University of Tennessee Center for Health Sciences. Men with oily hair should wash it every day, but avoid creamy shampoos that leave behind a heavy residue, which can weigh down oily hair. A postshampoo rinse with a solution of one teaspoon of vinegar in a pint of water can also help remove soap residues.

To the age-old question of whether to lather up and rinse once or twice when shampooing, there's no universal answer. In most cases, one round will do the trick; but if you have oily hair, work out-doors or live in a big city, you may have to suds up again to get your hair completely clean. Oily hair may need more cleaning in the sum-mer, when heat and humidity step up the production of sweat and oil on the scalp.

Shampooing is only the first step. To get hair really shiny, you need a conditioner. Conditioners contain ingredients that fill in nicks on the hair shaft and smooth the cuticle. They also cut down the amount of static in your hair. Static keeps hairs from lying smoothly together and allows them to tangle more readily, reducing shine. "Your hair naturally has a lot of negative ionic charges along the shaft," says Rebecca Caserio, M.D., clinical assistant professor of dermatology at the University of Pittsburgh. "This causes static. Conditioners add a positive charge, which helps neutralize the static."

"When the hairs lie together better," explains Dr. Corbett, "shine from one hair is reinforced by that of the adjacent hair. What the eye perceives as shine is actually groups of hairs lying parallel to one another to reflect the light."

Conditioners not only help protect hair from outside assaults, they also repair existing damage. But there are genuine differences among the ingredients used in conditioners. "If your hair is already damaged, it's especially important to choose a conditioner that will counteract the specific problem," says Dr. Corbett. For example, if your hair is very dry, try conditioners with small amounts of oil in them. (Look on the label for dimethicone or mineral oil.) For fine hair, select a conditioner with a watery consistency, such as a spray-on type that you leave on the hair.

There are two main ways to go about conditioning your hair: using a combination "conditioning shampoo," and using a separate conditioner. Conditioning shampoos, which combine the two func-tions in one product, work best for people whose hair isn't heavily damaged. (If you swim in pools a lot, work outdoors or live in a large city, that probably excludes you.) The advantage of conditioning shampoos is that they're convenient. The disadvantage is that they neither clean as well as plain cleansing shampoos nor condition as well as separate conditioners.

DO THICKENING SHAMPOOS WORK?

No shampoo or over-the-counter lotion can slow, halt or reverse hair loss. However, thickening shampoos and conditioners can make what you have *look* like more. They do this by coating hair shafts with balsam, polymers or proteins to make hair appear thicker; in some cases, they actually swell individual hairs. Look for terms like *body-building, thickening* or *volumizing* on the label.

These products are most effective for men whose hair is fine or in the early to middle stages of thinning. Try a few brands until you find one that seems to make a difference for you.

Some hair-styling aids, such as sprays, mousses and gel dressings, can also make hair look fuller, but beware of using them too often. They can make hair sticky, brittle and easy to break, which sort of defeats the purpose if you're already losing it.

A good compromise is to alternate. Try using a basic cleansing shampoo for every third or fourth washing and a conditioning shampoo the rest of the time.

Dry Facts about Dry Hair

If your hair is damaged, dry or prone to tangles, you probably need to use a separate conditioner all the time. Just remember that conditioners are formulated to cling to the hair shaft and not be rinsed away. With repeated use, this film can build up and attract dirt, leaving your hair looking limp. The problem is even worse if you use hair sprays and other styling aids, says Dr. Caserio. However, occasional use of a plain shampoo—and no conditioner—can keep this buildup from becoming a problem.

Another thing to look for is heat damage, so go easy with that blow dryer. Overdrying evaporates the water in the hair shaft that keeps it strong and pliable. To blow-dry for minimum damage and maximum shine:

• Towel-dry hair before you blow-dry. It's faster and easier on your hair.

• Use your blow dryer on a low heat setting.

• Hold it at least six inches from your head.

• Keep the dryer moving so the airflow isn't directed at the same spot for more than a few seconds.

• Gently finger-comb your hair while it's drying to prevent tangles.

• The top layer of your hair is particularly susceptible to overdrying because it takes the most abuse from the weather. Stop before this area is bone-dry.

That's all you need to know to keep your hair looking clean and shiny all the time . . . or should we say, to keep your *theoretical* hair clean and shiny all the time.

—William Harnham

Smooth Strokes

Avoiding razor nicks is a matter of sharp skills. Tape these tips on your bathroom mirror.

Al's beard is costing me money. At the poker table last week, I was thinking to myself that nothing's more irritating than trying to read his (formerly) expressive face now that he has this thick growth of ugly whiskers covering everything. I was looking at his up cards, wondering whether he'd pulled the case ace. Used to be, a little crease would form off to the side of his lip that would betray him. No more. I've had to resort to playing the cards.

In fairness to Al, however, maybe one thing's more irritating: the thing that brought on the beard in the first place. Turns out, a dermatologist told him he needed a beard to cure a bad case of ingrown hairs.

Technically, his condition is called pseudofolliculitis barbae, but "razor bumps" will do. It's the most common of many causes of inflamed hair follicles in men—especially black men. The painful bumps develop when the razor-sharpened tips of curly whiskers arc back to the skin and grow inward. "Once the hair comes back into the skin, it's attacked by the body's natural defenses just as any foreign body is, setting the stage for painful infections," says skin-care maven Lia Schorr, author of *Lia Schorr's Skin Care Guide for Men*.

One way to ward off the dreaded bumps is to do like Al and grow a beard, but that's rather extreme. Often a slight modification in your shaving regimen will do the trick. Men are encouraged to think a good shave means making the skin as smooth as a baby's behind, but the best thing for your skin may actually be *not* to shave that closely. "The closer you shave, the more you may encourage ingrown hairs, as only very short hairs can reenter the skin once they've come out," says Schorr.

These shaving tips may help prevent damage and keep things more comfortable.

Don't . . .

• Shave against the grain of your beard. This encourages hairs to be clipped below the skin's surface, where they can curve back and pierce the wall of the hair follicle.

• Stretch your skin taut while going over it with the blade. "When the skin is released, the short hairs pull back below the surface," says Jerome Litt, M.D., author of *Your Skin: From Acne to Zits*.

• Shave over an area more than twice. "No one will be examining your skin with a magnifying glass," says Schorr.

• Shave just before you exercise: Sweat irritates newly shaved skin.

Do . . .

• Go gently. A good shave doesn't have to do violence to your skin.

• Shave after showering so your face is as moist as possible. Otherwise, soak your beard for two minutes in hot, soapy water.

• Soften your face for two more minutes with shaving cream.

• Replace your blade often.

• Start at the upper cheeks and move down, thus exposing the beard's toughest areas to the cream's softening benefits longest.

Still, that's all preventive medicine. What if you've already got those nasty little bumps? Dr. Litt says you have to stop shaving for a few days at least. This gives the hairs that have looped back into your skin a chance to grow out—and it gives your skin a rest from the daily grind. Yes, the Don Johnson look went out a few years ago, but your skin doesn't care about fashion.

There is another alternative, but it's only for those who are truly dedicated. You can lift out those little ingrown-hair loops with a beard pick—a device with a sharp, curved tip—available at barber-supply stores. Try the Moore Technique Shaving System, designed by dermatologist Milton Moore, M.D. It comes with a preshave lubricant, anti-inflammatory cream, antibacterial cream and a beard pick. You'll find it at many pharmacies and some beauty salons—less than $20 for a two-month supply.

Dr. Litt also advises using a warm, wet washcloth to bring the bumps to a head, then plucking out the hairs with sterile tweezers. If you do this, yank in the direction of the growth. If you can't get it in two tries, give up: Digging around with the tweezers can irritate or inflame the skin. Al tried this approach and indeed found it made his skin more irritated. He was desperate, so he just grew the beard.

Fortunately, this wasn't a problem at his job, but it is for some men who grow beards and even for many who shave just every other day, says Robert Fitzpatrick, a Washington, D.C., attorney who cofounded the PFB (pseudofolliculitis barbae) Project "to fight job discrimination against bearded men." Fitzpatrick considers PFB a "societal disease" because pressure forces men with curly hair to shave clean.

Of course, rules about shaving aren't a problem if folliculitis crops up elsewhere on the body. Although razor bumps are the most common form of folliculitis, the pinhead-size yellow pustules can occur almost anywhere on the skin, says Richard Refowich, M.D., head of dermatology at St. Luke's Hospital in Bethlehem, Pennsylvania. For instance, they can result from bacteria picked up while soaking in hot tubs. Washing afterward with an antibacterial soap helps prevent infections. Topical antibiotics containing bacitracin or neomycin will usually clear them up, Dr. Refowich says.

I have another friend, Howie, who complains about ingrown hairs. I explained all the options. When I finally came to the easiest solution, he said, "No way." He's proud of his face, he told me. That was a month ago. Now his beard is making him uglier by the day.

—Richard Laliberte

Hide Your Hide

Who says there's no effortless way to slim down? Choosing the right wardrobe can make you look ten pounds lighter.

Forget about throwing your weight around at the office. In the business world, a pudgy profile makes you appear sloppy and disorganized—as though you lack self-control. In fact, studies show that thinner executives typically earn about $3,000 a year more than their heavier counterparts for doing the same work.

If you can't lose those stubborn extra few pounds, you still can avoid receiving a thinner paycheck by *looking* trimmer in the way you dress. Here's how.

Create vertical lines. Pinstripes are perfect. They draw the eye in a natural up-and-down direction, emphasizing height over width. Similarly, subtle or small patterns make you look taller than bold or big patterns, which break up the line of the body and seem to add bulk.

Dressing vertically also means wearing shirts and trousers that don't contrast. The eye stops at the boundary between a stark white shirt and black pants. Instead wear a gray shirt, so the vertical flow is uninterrupted.

Forget bow ties—that wide expanse of shirt underneath them just showcases your spare tire. Wear long ties, the tip of which should touch the top to middle of your belt. (A short tie resting on your stomach may prompt unwanted comparisons between you and Lou Costello.)

Wear cool colors. Black, charcoal gray and navy, aside from being classic suit colors that command authority, actually distance you from your observers and tend to unload some cargo. "Dark, cool, muted colors in a suit can make you appear 10 to 15 pounds slimmer," says image consultant Lois Fenton, author of *Dress for Excellence*. In sportswear, blue and green will also have slimming power. Conversely, steer clear of warm hues like red, yellow and orange. These colors bring you closer and bulk you up.

Beware of flashy clothes. For you, the sharkskin suit is a killing machine. Loud, shiny or bright colors draw all eyes to you and accentuate your width. If you love bright colors, save them for accents. It's fine to wear a tie and braces in startling hues. Under a gray or navy suit, a red or yellow tie will actually draw favorable attention to your face, fashion consultants say.

Wear light- to medium-weight fabrics. Heavyweight garments exaggerate girth. The best materials for a slimming effect: twills, gabardines and thin-wale corduroys. Leave bulky Harris tweeds to underfed professors.

Stay loose. Avoid close-fitting clothes; they emphasize bulges. It's particularly important that the upper chest, shoulders and upper sleeves of your jackets not be tight. Tight fabric there will stretch, wrinkle and bulge, producing a corrugated look.

Some final tips:

• If you're wide in the derriere, avoid ventless jackets. These tend to ride up in back, creating an effect about equal to wearing a sign that says "kick me." If your weight is in your torso, a ventless jacket can have a slimming effect, although some heavy men find ventless jackets less comfortable than those with center or side vents.

• Be careful with pleats. If they fit just right, pleated pants can hide a multitude of sins, but if you wear them too tight or if you're very large in the belly, the pleats will stand out, making you look like a fan. Generally, the wider the pleat, the less likely it is to spread apart.

• Cuffs tend to shorten legs and accentuate body width.

• For the beefy, barrel-chested man, the double row of buttons on double-breasted jackets cuts away thickness.

• Select shirts with button-down or standard collars rather than "wide load" spread collars.

—*Jennifer Whitlock*

Fill 'Er Up

Smile. When it comes to fixing cavities, picking the right fillin' isn't so chillin'. Here's some helpful information to chew on.

If you're like most guys, you don't have the slightest idea what kind of fillings your dentist puts in your mouth. He probably assumes you want the same type that's already in there, not realizing that when you had those teeth filled at 18, you were more interested in sneaking a peek at his assistant's cleavage than you were in what was going into that cavity in your third molar.

Well, you're a big boy now, and it's time you sat up in the dentist's chair and paid a little more attention. There's more than one way to fill a tooth. In fact, nowadays you have at least four choices: silver, gold, composite and porcelain. The following guide—plus a healthy dose of advice from your dentist—can help you decide which is right for you.

Silver

Silver is the workhorse of the bunch—it has been used far more often than any other filling material. And that's not surprising, since it was introduced more than 150 years ago. With that kind of history, it's no wonder dentists have a lot of faith in it. It's effective, easy for dentists to apply, and lasts for decades. It's also the least expensive of all the options.

Silver offers durability for high-stress areas like the back of the mouth, where biting force is greatest. It does tend to darken, though, so it may not be the best choice cosmetically for the front of the mouth.

These fillings are actually made from a combination of metals, including silver, copper, tin and mercury. The more proper name for this material is amalgam, but it's commonly called silver because of its color.

There is some controversy over the possibility that mercury might leak out of these fillings and harm people. (Mercury is toxic when ingested in high amounts.) At least one study has shown that mercury from silver fillings can cause kidney malfunction in test animals. The

209

American Dental Association (ADA), however, says there's "no reason for the public to be concerned."

A handful of dentists have tried to capitalize on the mercury scare by offering to replace silver fillings. Unless your fillings are cracked or discolored and need replacement, there's no reason to subject yourself to this. In fact, removing a mouthful of perfectly good fillings holds the potential for tooth damage.

Gold

Fillings made from this precious metal are also very durable, making it another good choice for the back of the mouth. Gold is especially useful for restoring teeth that have very large cavities. Such teeth are prone to cracking, and since gold fillings don't expand and contract with temperature changes as silver fillings do, they're less likely to cause a tooth to crack. In fact, gold is sometimes used to surround the outside of a tooth to prevent it from breaking. A softer filling, gold will not wear down the opposing teeth (as porcelain can). Finally, gold fillings last even longer than silver.

With this extra dependability, however, comes a bigger price tag. Depending on the size and location of the filling, gold can cost three to six times as much as silver. All of the extra cost may not be covered by your insurance, so you might want to check before you go for the gold.

Composite

These quartz/acrylic fillings are an appealing option for the front of your mouth because they can be colored to match your tooth enamel and blend in with your smile.

They haven't been around as long as gold and silver, though, so dentists aren't yet sure how long they last. The older composite fillings did have a tendency toward long-term "microleakage" (so small you can't see it), which could lead to decay under the filling. But the newer-generation composites bond more closely to the tooth and have much less of a leakage problem.

Composites are more susceptible to being worn down by opposing teeth, making them less desirable for back teeth. And solvents like alcohol and vinegar may weaken the composite.

For front teeth, the less durable but cosmetically agreeable composite may be a good choice. Composites are slightly more expensive than silver fillings.

Porcelain

Often lumped into a "white filling" category with composites, porcelain is actually a more durable cosmetic filling. Unlike composites, porcelain fillings do not wear down easily. But they are more abrasive toward opposing teeth than any other filling, "so your dentist may advise against them in areas where they would directly wear on other teeth or softer fillings," says Barry Dale, D.M.D., a spokesman for the Academy of General Dentistry.

Porcelain fillings are also more expensive than composites. Their higher price comes from the two-day procedure it takes to place them in the tooth. They're used most often in back teeth, especially those that show when you smile.

—Greg Gutfeld

New Lease on White

If flashing a high-beam smile is important to you, you're in luck. These at-home teeth-whitening kits can put the gleam back in your grin.

By the time a man reaches his midthirties, that blindingly white 150-watt smile he had when he was a kid has dimmed to about 75 watts or so. Even with diligent brushing, flossing and regular visits to the dental hygienist, teeth tend to yellow over the years as tiny interlacing cracks in the enamel absorb stains from coffee, tea, tobacco, wine and certain soft drinks.

It has been possible for some years now to bleach teeth back to their natural white color, but until recently that process involved three to five lengthy dental appointments (at $200 a shot) for teeth to be individually lightened. The dentist would cover your gums with a rubber guard, painstakingly apply a 30 percent hydrogen peroxide solution, Superoxol, to each tooth, and then blast it with a heat lamp to activate the bleach.

Today, in a technique some dentists are calling "revolutionary," you skip most of the office visits and bleach your own teeth. You start the program with a dental appointment to make sure your gums are healthy and your teeth clean. (The 10 percent carbamide peroxide solution or gel that's used can irritate unhealthy gums and won't work effectively on teeth with a lot of plaque buildup.) The dentist takes a mold of your teeth and creates a custom mouthpiece for you to take home. Each day you apply the peroxide gel to the mouthpiece and wear it for two to four hours.

Most people begin to see results in about a week, and the process is usually complete in a month. Twelve to 18 months down the line, you can use the mouthguard for a couple of hours just to keep the yellow at bay. Cost (including dentist visit and supplies): $150 to $500 per arch. Many people treat only the top teeth, as lowers aren't as prominent when you smile.

These dentist-supervised kits are catching on in a big way—at an American Dental Association (ADA) convention, about 90 percent of the 500 dentists attending a lecture on the subject said they were using the mouthpiece technique. Only about 2 to 3 percent said they were having problems with it.

Over-the-Counter Kits

For a much less expensive alternative, there are many over-the-counter teeth whiteners. These pastes or polishes may contain weaker concentrations of some kind of peroxide agent than dentist-supervised kits and are designed to be left on the teeth for as little as ten minutes per day.

But there's not much hard evidence on how well they work. Some patients report favorable, though unpredictable, results with mild stains. "Little research exists on the long-term safety of these products, but as yet, few problems have been reported," says Joel M. Boriskin, D.D.S., chief of the Division of Dentistry at Highland General Hospital, Oakland, California.

Still, dentists will tend to steer you away from the do-it-yourself kits. Chakwan Siew, Ph.D., head of the ADA's Department of Toxicology, warns that long-term use of hydrogen peroxide can damage chromosomes and boost the cancer-causing effects of other substances. Peroxide may also infect or damage the soft tissues of the mouth or even the interior of the tooth. (None of that is likely if you stay within the product guidelines.)

Some over-the-counter kits include their own mouthguard. But Richard Price, D.M.D., a consumer advisor for the ADA, warns that an ill-fitting mouthguard could actually hold the bleach against the gums and burn them—precisely the problem it is designed to prevent. The mouthguard needs to be custom fitted and trimmed, he says—"One size does not fit all."

But several manufacturers of at-home bleaching kits, notably EpiSmile and Den-Mat (makers of the Rembrandt Lighten system), are cooperating with the ADA. In a study reported in the *Journal of Esthetic Dentistry,* the Rembrandt system produced a "definite improvement relative to the shade of the treated teeth" in 43 patients and left "no sensitivity or unpleasant aftertaste."

In the Dentist's Office

A follow-up study found no complications and in some cases an *improvement* in the condition of the gums.

If bleaching isn't doing the trick for you or isn't appropriate, con-sider these teeth-whitening options.

Bonding. In this procedure, your teeth are covered with a paste-like bonding material that's hardened under high-intensity light. It lasts from three to eight years. Cost: $200 to $500 per tooth.

Veneers. The front of the tooth is painted with adhesive, then an ultrathin porcelain veneer is pressed into place. At $275 to $850 per tooth, this is more expensive than composite bonding, but veneers can last for ten years or more.

Crowns. Capping a tooth with a crown may be the only option for severe stains. Crowns require more work and are more expensive than veneers. They last 10 to 12 years. Cost: $445 to $1,000 per tooth.

—Ron Heitzgebot

Optical Options

Confused by all the styles and choices when you shop for eyeglasses? Here's a buyer's guide to help you see your way clear.

Let me describe my typical visit to an eyeglass store. I step through the door of Lens Land or Optical World or whatever and immediately I am confronted by four million sets of frames hanging on invisible racks. I'm still trying to figure out which are the men's and which are the ladies' when an attractive woman approaches and asks if I need help.

"Uh, yes," I reply. "I need some new glasses."

"Great. Are you interested in metal frames or plastic? Single vision or bifocals? Glass or polycarbonate lenses? Scratch-resistant coating? Antireflective tint? UV filtering?"

At this point I reach for my checkbook and turn my decisions completely over to the salesperson. A few weeks later I stop back to pick up my glasses and return home, whereupon my girlfriend says something like, "Hmmm. New glasses. Um, maybe you should take me with you next time you get new frames."

Sound at all familiar?

These days, buying prescription eyeglasses is a real challenge. You're faced with considerable (and often confusing) options on everything from the size of the frame to the types of lenses and what they're coated with. At least when you shop for a car, you get to take a test drive and kick the tires. With glasses you're stuck with the choices you make up front.

I've found that shopping for eyeglasses is a lot easier when you're armed with some basic information. Whether you get your next pair from a private optician or optometrist or at that flashy optical chain at the mall, it pays to do a little homework. To help, I've assembled a summary of what's out there in vision wear, including materials, coatings and lenses. Take a look.

Lens Material

Glass. All eyeglasses used to have glass lenses, and it remains a popular material, mainly because it provides a hard, scratch-resistant surface. Its big drawback is its weight.

"If you have a high-powered prescription, wearing thick glass lenses may be too much weight for your nose to bear," says Irving Bennett, O.D., of the American Optometric Association.

Plastic. "Plastic lenses are safer, more impact-resistant and much lighter than glass, giving you a more comfortable fit," says Richard Morgenthal, of Morgenthal-Frederics Opticians, in New York City. When larger lenses became fashionable, lightweight plastic came to dominate the market. However, plastic lenses are much more vulnerable to scratches than glass. "You should always get a scratch-resistant coating on your plastic lenses," says Dr. Bennett. Some places may offer the coating as standard with plastic lenses.

Polycarbonate plastic. These lenses are made of a lighter but tougher plastic distinctive enough that eye-care specialists classify them in a separate category. Polycarbonate-plastic lenses were first introduced as virtually unbreakable, with people slamming hammers on them to show off the lenses' strength. Experts say most people don't really need this kind of protection. Polycarbonate is recommended for children younger than 16 and anyone who plays contact sports or who works in a hazardous industry. Polycarbonate, although strong, is still prone to scratching, so if you choose it, get the scratch-resistant coating.

Coatings and Filters

While coatings are becoming an increasingly popular extra, the real need for some may be overstated. Also, they don't last forever. Most opticians agree that if you take really good care of coated lenses, clean them carefully and don't wipe them on your shirttail, coatings can last a few years.

Scratch-resistant coatings. As the name implies, these don't make plastic lenses scratchproof, but they do protect against the hairline scratches that occur from normal cleaning and handling. They won't prevent damage from more serious indiscretions such as throwing your glasses on the car dash, dropping them on the sidewalk or putting them in the same pocket as your car keys.

If you buy glass lenses, you won't need this coating. It is necessary for polycarbonate lenses and recommended for plastic ones.

Tints. Tints, especially the colors brown, green and gray, may help give you clearer vision in sunlight. If you opt for a tint, make sure it's not so dark that it impairs your vision indoors.

UV filters. Most glasses these days already come with built-in protection from ultraviolet rays. "The majority of UV light is filtered by any glass or plastic material," says H. Jay Wisnicki, M.D., director of ophthalmology at Beth Israel Medical Center in New York City. "The extra coatings may not be that important." Take the windows of your car, for example. If you drive with your arm against the window in the blistering sun, it won't get burned. But hang it out the window and you may get a truck-driver's tan. That's the kind of protection you get with most glass. If you want extra peace of mind, you can opt for the coating, but it's not really needed, says Dr. Wisnicki.

As for UV rays seeping from computers, that threat, too, may be exaggerated. "The amount of UV light that comes from a computer is very small and shouldn't be regarded as a problem," says Dr. Wisnicki. The American Academy of Ophthalmology considers video display terminals (VDTs) to be completely safe, presenting no hazard to the eye.

Photochromic lenses. Photochromics, lenses that change from clear to dark, may be a convenient choice for someone whose job requires a combination of indoor and outdoor work. Different brands go from light when indoors to varying degrees of darkness when outside. "They shouldn't be used for driving, however, because the lenses need UV light to stimulate darkening, and UV light is blocked by windshield glass," says Morgenthal.

If you have photochromics, here's a tip to make them work better: "If you consistently store these lenses overnight in the refrigerator, they'll respond quicker to light and get darker," says Morgenthal.

Antireflective coatings. This coating—made from the same material used to coat camera lenses and binoculars—can block out reflected glare. Consider it if you do a lot of night driving—it virtually eliminates the starburst effect you get from oncoming headlights. It can also cut glare from other types of lighting.

One of the drawbacks of antiglare coating, though, is a tendency to smudge. You'll have to take extra care to keep your lenses clean. Dr. Wisnicki, who owns a pair, agrees, saying, "The dirt seems to show up more." There's a new Teflon-like coating out now, though, that goes over the antiglare coating and may make the lenses easier to care for.

Special Lenses

High-index lenses. These are simply denser lenses with a higher power of refraction, meaning they can bend more light than standard-index glasses, so less material is needed to do the job. Thus the lenses can be thinner and lighter.

They're a must for anyone who needs strong prescription glasses but who doesn't want the Coke-bottle look.

Bifocals. Previously, when it came to combating presbyopia (the gradual decline in the eye lens's ability to focus on nearby objects), one could turn only to bifocals. With them, only two distances mattered—near and far. There was no in between. Now new lenses offer effective alternatives to the split-level world of bifocal vision, some that erase the bifocals' age-giveaway lines while giving sharp vision at different distances.

Trifocals. Bifocals have the "near" and "far" covered. Trifocals offer an extra area of power on the lens to bridge the near and far. The visual breakdown when looking through a common trifocal lens goes like this: far distance up top, medium distance in the middle and close at the bottom.

Trifocals aren't for everyone. "Some people may not be able to get used to the 'image jumps' that occur when switching from one segment to the next," says Richard E. Lippman, O.D., director of the Division of Ophthalmic Devices for the Food and Drug Administration. It's a problem encountered with bifocals and can become more troublesome in a trifocal with the extra segment, he says.

Progressive-addition lenses. If the bifocal or trifocal is the stairway of lenses, then a progressive bifocal lens is the smooth ramp. Gone are the abrupt jumps in vision power. You see a blended transition from one segment of vision to the next, closely mimicking good natural vision.

The most obvious benefit the progressive-addition lenses have over bifocals is the absence of the age-telling demarcation lines—the lines can't be seen because the focal powers blend into each other.

Ready-to-wears. You've seen them in neat racks at the pharmacy—simple reading glasses that cost about $12 a pair. They're inexpensive, but are they a good idea for poor eyesight?

"When it comes to reading newspapers or other types of short-term reading, these glasses are harmless," says Dr. Lippman. However, he adds a caveat: "Because these lenses come in basic, fixed corrections, with no gradual increments in between, you're really guessing at your prescription when you pick one up," he says. "They shouldn't keep you from getting regular checkups to determine what kind of correction you need and to see if there's any underlying illness behind the vision change."

Pricing

Every company that sells eyeglasses has its own pricing system. Some charge the same for plastic and glass lenses, while others may charge more for one than the other. Some offer options like free tints, while others tack on $15 to $30 extra. So what do you do and where do you start?

"Be wary of come-ons and promotions," warns Dr. Bennett. Those buy-one-pair-get-one-free spiels, for example. "They usually involve a discontinued product," he says. "It'll be a naked lens with no frills, coatings or treatments—and they may nail you on that."

Don't be surprised if you find that the major chains—the ones found most frequently at malls—charge a little more. "Having a sales force, paying higher rent and using expensive machinery makes their overhead higher, so it's understandable their prices are higher," says Dr. Bennett.

The key, then, is to get an idea of what you want beforehand and call around. If you feel you're getting a sales pitch instead of honest advice, skip the place. Compare identical products. A plastic lens with a scratch-resistant coating and a gray tint may be priced differently from one with high-index and antiglare coating.

Ask for itemized prices for all the lenses and coatings, and be sure you're comparing the same brands. And don't forget money-back guarantees. Many brands of lenses and coatings carry them. It's up to you to ask.

I've found, or rather my girlfriend has reminded me, that it's hard to judge for yourself what kind of frames look best on your face. My favorite glasses are some snazzy oval tortoiseshells. I see them on men all the time and I like the way they look. But on me, according to my significant other, they look stupid.

If you're not sure what kind of frames you look best in, bring along a friend to help you decide. Don't rely on the salesperson. She's probably been asked that question 200 times that day and is beyond rational judgment.

—Greg Gutfeld

Timely Contacts

Extended-wear contact lenses are great, as long as you don't take the "extended" part too literally. How long can you leave your new lenses in?

If you sleep with your extended-wear contact lenses in, you're 10 to 15 times more likely to develop a painful and potentially serious eye condition called ulcerative keratitis than people who take their lenses out every night, reports a team of ophthalmologists from the Massachusetts Eye and Ear Infirmary and Harvard Medical School.

"I wouldn't tell most people that they should never sleep with their contact lenses in, but they certainly should never do it for more than seven days," warns Johanna M. Seddon, M.D., one of the researchers.

Ulcerative keratitis occurs when an abrasion in the cornea, the clear covering of the eye, allows bacteria to enter and cause an infection. Untreated, it can impair sight by causing scar tissue to form, blocking part of the field of vision.

Until about a decade ago, virtually all cases of ulcerative keratitis occurred in eyes that were already predisposed somehow to such damage, says Dr. Seddon. But as soft contact lenses became popular, eye doctors began seeing it in eyes that were otherwise healthy. Contact lenses now account for about 30 percent of the cases. And most of those, says Dr. Seddon, can be blamed on excessive overnight lens wearing.

Exactly how is still unknown. But there are some clues. "Contact lenses can cause tiny injuries to the cornea, and they also reduce the amount of oxygen that reaches it," she says. "Both factors could let bacteria and other harmful organisms establish themselves."

It turns out that extended-wear lens users aren't the only people who go to bed without taking out their contacts. In the Harvard study, the doctors found a surprising number of *daily*-wear lens users did. And as you might expect, they, too, had an increased incidence of ulcerative keratitis.

"I have to emphasize that it's not contact lenses that are the risk factor here," says Dr. Seddon. "The risky thing is leaving them in for several days in a row."

Rules to Live By

When extended-wear contacts came on the market, the Food and Drug Administration allowed manufacturers to say they could be left in for 30 days between cleanings. Partly as a result of the new study, the month is now down to 7 days. Some eye doctors say it should be shortened even more. Dr. Seddon suggests sleeping with your lenses out at least once or twice a week to be safe. "The results of our study suggest that your risk of ulceration increases 5 percent every night you sleep with extended-wear lenses in," she says.

Dr. Seddon and her colleagues found that the other major risk factor for ulcerative keratitis was lens hygiene—or, more specifically, the lack of it. "The overall level of lens care was alarmingly low" in everyone they studied, the doctors wrote. When you're cleaning your lenses, don't overlook the case you keep them in. "The lens case should be scrubbed clean with water every other day or so," Dr. Seddon says.

We shouldn't have to make this last point, but the medical researchers say we do: There is one thing that all eye doctors agree no one should *ever* do, and that's put a lens in your mouth!

—*Martha Capwell*

High-Tech Socks

Want to be blister-free at last? Invest a few bucks in the latest style foot protection and you'll never blister again.

For so many of us, the thrill of working out is all too often muted by the agony of the feet. That's because when it comes to selecting athletic footgear, many men concentrate on shoes but overlook the socks. Yes, socks.

According to Wayne Axman, D.P.M., a New York triathlete who is also a sports podiatrist, men will spend hours poring over shoe guides, comparing information on the midsoles and cushioning properties of basketball, tennis, running and hiking shoes, and then plunk down a C note and some change for a high-tech model. But when it comes to socks, they go no-tech and rummage through their drawers for anything handy.

Guilty as charged. I used to be like that. I always mixed the latest in shoe technology with cheapo socks. Not only was my sock collection thin—as in socks worn and frayed in the heel and toe-box areas—but at times I even played full-court hoops sockless if I couldn't round up a pair of socks at game time.

Times have changed and so have I. Instead of wearing the same socks for cycling, basketball and running, my particular sport passions, I now wear different types of socks for each. The sport-specific socks now found in athletic stores are more than just filler for your shoes, more than covering for the feet. They're integral pieces of sports equipment, just like your shoes. Materials such as polypropylene, Lycra, spandex, high-bulk acrylic, CoolMax and Thermax have been added to socks, almost eliminating natural fibers.

Real Comfort from Synthetics

Some podiatrists say these new synthetic socks are better for you than the old standbys like cotton or wool. It all has to do with wicking, the ability of synthetics to effectively move perspiration from the foot. "Yes, cotton socks may initially feel comfortable when you put them on," says Rosario J. La Barbera, D.P.M., past president of the American Podiatric Medical Association, "but once you run a few miles in cotton socks or play a set of tennis in them, the sweat buildup remains with the fabric. And that's what leads to blisters, thickened toenails and fungal infections."

"Socks that are made of 100 percent acrylic or blends of natural and synthetic fibers are the way to go," agrees Douglas H. Richie, D.P.M., a Seal Beach, California, podiatrist whose sock tests at the Long Beach Marathon confirmed that runners in synthetic-based socks suffered fewer blisters than those wearing cotton socks.

Synthetic fibers also retain their shape and texture longer. After a few machine washings, cotton socks without the added resilient synthetics become limp and shapeless. Synthetics tend to bounce back to their original shape. One caution: Bleach can damage synthetic fibers. Wash as directed.

Beyond the new materials, the very construction of socks is different today. Basketball socks have a high heel cushion to minimize pressure from the sneaker heel. Tennis socks come with ribbed insteps to help dissipate lace pressure. Ski socks come with reinforced shin shields to protect against "boot bang." In addition, there are specialty socks made for mountain-bike riding, walking, fishing, hiking, golf, snowboarding, soccer and baseball, many of them with added shock absorption to protect your feet from the wear and tear of running. "When you run, each footfall brings down approximately two to three times your body weight on your foot," Dr. Axman says. "A good pair of athletic shoes, along with well-padded socks, will absorb a lot of that pounding."

Let's look at the advantages, sock by sock.

All-Purpose

Double Lay-R Cross Trail Fitness Sock has Kevlar (the same material used in bulletproof vests) added to the toes and heel for extra durability.

Ridgeview CoolMax Cross-Trainer is lightweight and made with an exclusive channel fiber to wick perspiration away from the skin.

PrimaSport Crew offers a fully cushioned forefoot to minimize foot impact in running and jumping, and Bioguard, a special odor killer that's said to last the life of the socks.

Running

Nike CoolMax Run/Cycle Sock is a sleek, totally cushionless sock that fits like a glove and is recommended for those who want to feel the technical features of their shoes.

PrimaSport Wicking Quarter Top is another synthetic blend designed to keep your feet dry.

Ridgeview CoolMax Running Sock is excellent for perspiration control. The CoolMax fiber is a synthetic that is superior for wicking sweat away.

Thor-Lo JMX Mini-Crew features an extrathick, spongy impact zone at the ball and heel, with lower-density padding at the arch so the sock doesn't bunch up.

Thor-Lo RMX is a midweight designed for racers that offers even more shock absorption, while the stretch nylon instep provides a "sockless" feel.

Biking

Brilliant CoolMax will keep your feet cool and dry, and the colors will make you hard to miss.

Double Lay-R ATB 54 is for the serious mountain-bike rider. Both toe and heel are reinforced with Kevlar for durability. The sock has a black cuff so dirt stains won't be a problem.

Performance Pro Line socks combine high-wicking CoolMax and special vented side panels for improved breathability.

PrimaSport CoolMax Quarter Top uses CoolMax fiber for perspiration control and a Spandex top to keep the socks from rolling down.

Thor-Lo CMC is an ultrathin sock that's padded in the heel and ball for shock absorption and has CoolMax to draw off the sweat.

Racket Sports

Nike Court Crew blends CoolMax with cotton to offer a sock that protects against friction during lateral court movement.

PrimaSport Court CoolMax Quarter Top offers what they call a Landing Pad cushioning system, which uses ribbing in the sole and toe for shock absorption and to prevent foot slide.

Ridgeview Tennis Sock features Duraspun, a synthetic fiber that provides bulk and cushioning for maximum shock absorption, along with good perspiration wicking.

Thor-Lo Tennis Crew TX blends acrylic and nylon fibers and is thickly padded at the ball and heel, with a pad over the toe to protect against skin abrasion.

Basketball

PrimaSport over the Calf offers special calf support.

Ridgeview Basketball Sock, used by many NBA players, offers high-bulk Duraspun fiber for extra shock absorption.

Thor-Lo BX Basketball Sock features an extended heel pad to protect the Achilles tendon.

Hiking

Double Lay-R Lightweight Field Combo Pak actually consists of two different socks, a CoolMax boot liner to wick moisture away from the foot and an outer sock of polypropylene, nylon and wool that you wear over the liner. It is guaranteed to keep your feet blister-free.

PrimaSport Thermax over the Calf combines Thermax and wool for superior warmth during cool- and cold-weather hiking, fishing and mountaineering.

Thor-Lo KX Hiking Crew Sock is padded in the heel and the ball of the foot to protect against blisters and abrasion. Use them for day trips or easy overnights when you're not carrying too much weight.

—*Gerald Couzens*

PART 9

Bod Like a Rock

Make Gains Fast

Get the ultimate workout in just 40 minutes. Dozens of top exercise experts tell you how to squeeze the most pump into the least amount of time.

If you want stronger muscles, a better body and more speed and endurance but aren't doing anything to get them, we bet we know why: no time. There's the job, the business trips, the family, the friends, the yard chores, the civic club, the newspapers and trade journals. You have the best of intentions, but you also have a very full dance card.

Well, we're here to say you can make your fitness goals and have a life, too. All you have to do is find a measly 40 minutes, three times a week. That's long enough to get your heart and muscles pumping and short enough to stave off boredom, and it fits neatly into a lunch hour with some time to spare.

The secret of fast fitness is efficiency. *Men's Health* consulted dozens of top exercise physiologists, coaches and professional athletes to help us create short, targeted workouts for every man—whether your goal is muscle growth, weight loss or general fitness.

Consistency is the key to success. You'll get the fastest results if you follow a Monday-Wednesday-Friday routine. "A man begins to lose the strength and endurance benefits he's gained from his exercise program after 60 hours away from the gym," says Charles Kuntzleman, Ed.D., national program director for Fitness Finders. "But even a two-day-a-week program is better than no program at all."

Each of these workout programs should begin with a warm-up and end with a cool-down. The warm-up—essentially some calisthenics or light aerobic activity like brisk walking or stationary cycling, followed by some stretching—allows your muscles, heart and lungs to ease into the session without shocking your system. The cool-down takes your body back to a resting state more gradually. When you stop short, your heart rate and blood pressure plummet, which can cause feelings of light-headedness or dizziness. Winding down slowly also helps to clear lactic acid, a by-product of intense exercise, out of your bloodstream. Some experts believe that lactic acid is responsible for delayed-onset muscle soreness—that achy feeling that strikes the day after a workout. Stretching is also important; it keeps muscles limber and reduces the risk of injury.

For guidance on the correct form for the exercises that follow, check with the fitness instructor at your health club, try a session with a personal trainer, or check out one of these books: *Getting Stronger,* by Bill Pearl and Gary T. Moran; *The Complete Book of Nautilus Training,* by Michael D. Wolf; and *Home Gym Fitness: Free Weight Workouts,* by Charles T. Kuntzleman.

Before starting, you'll need to know a few numbers. First figure out your maximum heart rate (max H.R.): max H.R. = 220 − your age. Next determine your correct heart-rate training range. This depends on your exercise goals.

For example, a 40-year-old man on the Fat Burner program would first calculate his maximum heart rate (220 − 40 = 180); then he would look up the desired training range for that workout. In his case, it's 60 to 70 percent of his maximum heart rate. So to get the desired benefits, he should try to keep his heart rate between 108 (0.60 × 180) and 126 (0.70 × 180) beats per minute.

To calculate your pulse rate, press lightly with two fingers on your wrist or neck, count the number of beats you feel in 10 seconds and multiply that number by 6. For constant feedback on your intensity level, try a heart-rate monitor. The new models are an amazingly accurate and reasonably priced way to keep tabs on your workouts—some models even offer computer hookups that allow you to graph your fitness progress.

Here are our programs. (Do check with your doctor before proceeding.)

General Fitness Routine

This plan is perfect for the man who's just starting to exercise or who doesn't have any specific exercise goals other than to look and feel better. It provides a solid strength and endurance base. If you're out of shape, you should start here, even though competing in the Ironman may be your ultimate goal. After about eight weeks on this program, you'll be ready to start one of the more advanced ones.

MONDAY AND FRIDAY

Start: Warm-up #1 (see "Warm-Ups" on page 232), 5 minutes.

Middle: Fifteen minutes of continuous aerobic exercise (60 to 70 percent of max H.R.) such as brisk walking, running, biking, stair climbing, cross-country skiing or rowing, followed by 15 minutes of weight training using either machines or free weights.

Do the exercises below in order, in a circuit fashion—performing one complete set of eight to ten repetitions and then moving to the next. Rest 30 seconds between stations. In 15 minutes, you should be able to do two complete circuits. For each machine, start with a weight that allows you to do ten easy repetitions. Once you're comfortable with your form, increase the weight (one notch or plate on exercise machines, five pounds with free weights) every other workout until you reach the maximum weight you can lift for that exercise and still complete ten repetitions for each of two sets.

Exercise Stations: Leg extension, leg curl, low back machine, bench press, lat pulldown, military press, tricep pushdown, bicep curl.

Finish: Cool-down #1 (see "Cool-Downs" on page 233), 5 minutes.

WEDNESDAY

Start: Warm-up #1 (see "Warm-Ups" on page 232), 5 minutes.

Middle: A 30-minute aerobic circuit. This should be done just like the circuit program on Monday and Friday, with a single significant exception: *Replace the 30 seconds of rest between sets with 30 seconds of aerobic exercise.* For example, when you get off the bench press machine, immediately hop on a stationary cycle, jump rope or run in place before moving on to flies. Eliminating the rest period and adding aerobic activity between sets allows you to get an aerobic workout while weight lifting. Do two circuits, each consisting of the following exercises.

Exercise Stations: Leg extension, leg press, leg curl, calf raise, low back machine or hyperextensions, push-up, bench press, fly, military press, lateral raises, upright row, pull-up, lat pulldown, tricep pushdown, bicep curl.

Finish: Cool-down #1 (see "Cool-Downs" on page 233), 5 minutes.

The Fat Burner

Got a couple of stubborn pounds sitting around your midsection that you'd like to lose? This is the program for you. Burning fat is actually easier than most people think. It doesn't require long, painful hours in the gym or the humiliation of being wrapped in plastic and trundled off to a steam room. "Consistency and moderate aerobic exercise are the keys to losing weight," says Stu Mittleman, a personal trainer and owner of New York Ultrafit, a center for fitness evaluations and personal training. "Choose exercises that you enjoy and can sustain for 20 to 30 minutes of continuous activity three times a week."

MONDAY AND FRIDAY

Start: Warm-up #1 (see "Warm-Ups" on page 232), 5 minutes.

Middle: Thirty minutes of continuous aerobic exercise (60 to 70 percent of max H.R.) such as brisk walking, running, biking, stair climbing, cross-country skiing or rowing.

Finish: Cool-down #2 (see "Cool-Downs" on page 233), 5 minutes.

WEDNESDAY

Start: Warm-up #1 (see "Warm-Ups" on page 232), 5 minutes.

Middle: Thirty minutes of aerobic exercise (60 to 75 percent of max H.R.). Switch exercises every 5 to 10 minutes. For example, do 5 minutes on the stationary bike, 5 minutes on the rowing machine, 5 minutes on the treadmill, 5 minutes on the stair climber, 5 minutes on the cross-country ski machine, 5 minutes jumping rope. (If you don't have a wide variety of equipment available, alternate between bench stepping, rope jumping and jogging in place.)

Finish: Cool-down #2 (see "Cool-Downs" on page 233), 5 minutes.

Endurance Builder

To increase endurance, you'll have to turn up the volume. "Moderately paced exercise is fine for burning calories, but when you want to build your endurance, you have to work at a slightly higher intensity level," says Budd Coates, exercise physiologist and world-class marathoner. "Over time, your cardiovascular system adapts to the added stress, making you more efficient and letting you go longer and farther with less effort."

MONDAY, WEDNESDAY AND FRIDAY

Start: Warm-up #1 (see "Warm-Ups" on page 232), 5 minutes.

Middle: Thirty minutes of continuous aerobic exercise (70 to 80 percent of max H.R.). Use any exercises you like, such as brisk walking, running, biking, stair climbing, cross-country skiing or rowing, so long as you maintain your target heart rate.

You may use different machines on different days, but remain on one machine during a single exercise session. It's very difficult to maintain an intensity level of 70 to 80 percent of max H.R. while changing machines.

If you can't stay at this level for the full 30 minutes (and you won't be able to at first), it's okay to reduce the intensity until you get your breath back (about 3 minutes). Then if you feel better, up the intensity to your target zone. Use as many recovery slowdowns as you need to get through the 30 minutes, but keep going and keep trying to get your heart rate back up into the training range. As your body adapts, your endurance will improve, and you will need fewer breaks.

Finish: Cool-down #2 (see "Cool-Downs" on page 233), 5 minutes.

Speed Builder

In a hurry? Whether you're preparing for a race or just looking to get a step ahead of the competition in your racquetball game, this workout's for you. Its high intensity not only gets results but also gets them fast. In fact, this is the one workout where we're going to tell you to cut your session short. Go for the burn. Then get back to your office. You can be done in much less time than 40 minutes.

"When you're talking speed or increased performance, you need intervals," says Pat Croce, physical conditioning coach for the Philadelphia Flyers and 76ers. Intervals are repeated short periods of intense exercise (like wind sprints) broken up by light exercise (like jogging in place or bench stepping) for recovery.

MONDAY AND FRIDAY

Follow Monday and Friday "Endurance Builder" program schedule exactly as described. (See page 229.)

WEDNESDAY

Start: Warm-up #2 (see "Warm-Ups" on page 232), 10 minutes.

Middle: Five sets consisting of one minute of hard aerobic activity (80 to 90 percent of max H.R.) followed by one minute of very easy aerobic activity to recover. Some suggested activities: running, race walking, biking, stair climbing, cross-country skiing or rowing.

Finish: Cool-down #3 (see "Cool-Downs" on page 233), 10 minutes.

Muscle Toner

Not all bodybuilders want to look like the Wild Samoan. This program is for a man who seeks more strength and vitality but an overall appearance that's lean and firm, not brawny. Building muscle tone is a careful process of shaping—some might even say sculpting—the muscles. The result is a subtle increase in what bodybuilders call "definition"—the ripple effect. It's a two-pronged effort: part fat burning, part muscle building.

MONDAY AND FRIDAY

Start: Warm-up #3 (see "Warm-Ups" on page 232), 5 minutes.

Middle: Thirty minutes of weight training, using free weights whenever possible. "When building muscle tone, it is important to use lighter weights and do fast-paced repetitions with little rest between sets," says Anthony D. Mahon, Ph.D., of Ball State's Human Performance Laboratory. Use a circuit approach, going from one machine to the next fairly quickly. The rapid pace adds fat-burning aerobic benefits.

Do the exercises below in order. On each machine, crank out 10 to 12 repetitions, rest 30 seconds and then move to the next station. In 30 minutes, you should be able to do two complete circuits. Start with a weight that allows you to do 12 easy repetitions. Once you're comfortable with your form, increase the weight 5 to 10 pounds every other workout until you can do 12 repetitions of the exercise on the first circuit but only 10 on the second. Once your muscles adapt to this new weight and you can blast out 12 repetitions on both circuits, bump the weight up another notch.

Exercise Stations: Leg extension, leg press, leg curl, calf raise, low back machine, bench press with barbell or dumbbells, dumbbell fly, lat pulldown behind the head, military press with barbell or dumbbells, seated row with cables or machine, lateral raise with dumbbells, upright row with barbell or dumbbells, tricep pushdown on machine, bicep curl with barbell or dumbbells, wrist curl with barbell or dumbbells.

Finish: Cool-down #1 (see "Cool-Downs" on page 233), 5 minutes.

WEDNESDAY

Start: Warm-up #3 (see "Warm-Ups" on page 232), 5 minutes.

Middle: A 30-minute circuit program as on Monday and Friday, but with a few modifications. This workout contains fewer exercises, giving you time to do three circuits instead of two. Also, whereas the Monday and Friday workouts concentrate on free weights, this workout uses machines. Changing to machines will work your muscles at slightly different angles, producing a wider range of strength and better definition. Perform three circuits of 10 to 12 repetitions of each of the following exercises, allowing yourself 30 seconds of rest between sets. Set out all the dumbbells and barbells you need before you start so you can move through your workout with no unnecessary delay.

Exercise Stations: Leg extension, leg curl, low back machine, bench press on machine, fly on machine, lat pulldown to chest, military press on machine, lateral raise on machine, tricep kickback, bicep curl on machine.

Finish: Cool-down #1 (see "Cool-Downs" on page 233), 5 minutes.

Body Blaster

Size has its benefits. Let's face it: Larger men seem to have a more dominating presence in the world. If you want to make sure nobody ever kicks sand in your face at the beach, this is your program.

Here, the rhythm is quite different from all the other workouts. The pace slows down, and the focus is on volume (pounds lifted) not intensity (speed of the repetitions). "When building muscle, you want to concentrate on overloading the muscle, so you have to use heavier weights than you would if you were going for tone," says Frank Zane, three-time Mr. Universe and three-time Mr. Olympia turned personal trainer.

WARM-UPS

To help ready your muscles for more strenuous activity, do these warm-ups as indicated in the exercise routines described in this chapter.

Warm-up #1

Use this warm-up for all aerobic-related routines.

• Three minutes of gentle aerobic exercise, doing a scaled-down version of the activity you'll perform in the main part of the routine. For example, if you're going to run, walk briskly or jog; if you're going to use the stair climber, set the machine about half as high as you will during the main part of the exercise.

• Two minutes of stretching, concentrating on the muscles you're going to use or on those that feel especially tight. For example, if you're going to ride a bike, pay particular attention to your quads and your lower back; if you plan to run, key on hamstrings and calves.

Warm-up #2

• Three minutes of gentle aerobic exercise, doing a scaled-down version of the same activity you'll perform in the main part of the routine.

• Two minutes of stretching, concentrating on the muscles you're going to use in the main part of the workout.

• Five minutes of moderate aerobic activity such as brisk walking, running, biking, stair climbing, cross-country skiing or rowing.

Warm-up #3

• Three minutes of calisthenics, consisting of two sets of push-ups and two sets of sit-ups or crunches.

• Two minutes of stretching, concentrating on the muscles you're going to use or on those that feel especially tight. Note: Stretching can be done between sets to loosen up particular muscles before or after they have been worked.

COOL-DOWNS

Cool-down is an important component of any workout; be sure to do these routines as advised in this chapter.

Cool-down #1

• Two sets of sit-ups or crunches.

• Three minutes of stretching, concentrating on muscles worked in the session or on those that feel especially tight.

Cool-down #2

• Two minutes of gentle aerobic exercise, doing a scaled-down version of the same activity performed in the main part of the routine.

• One set of sit-ups or crunches.

• One set on low back machine.

• Two minutes of stretching, concentrating on muscles worked in the session or on those that feel especially tight.

Cool-down #3

• Five minutes of moderate aerobic activity—whatever you were doing in the main part of the routine.

• Five minutes of stretching.

Further, when size is your goal, it is best to work one body part at a time instead of following a circuit program, so you can really overload the muscle and encourage the most growth. Do all three sets of one exercise before moving on to the next. Take your time. The slow pace will also allow you more rest between sets—and you'll need it so your body can recover for another intense effort.

MONDAY AND FRIDAY

Start: Warm-up #3 (see "Warm-Ups" on page 232), 5 minutes.

Middle: A 30-minute weight-training program as described under Muscle Toner on page 230. Do three sets of each exercise, resting 45 seconds to 1 minute between sets. Increase the weight and decrease the repetitions with each set. On the first set, do 8 to 12 repetitions; on the second, do 6 to 8; on the third, you should be able to complete only 3 to 6.

Exercise Stations: Leg extension, leg press, bench press with barbell or dumbbells, lat pulldown behind the head, military press with barbell, upright row with barbell, tricep pushdown on machine, bicep curl with barbell.

Finish: Cool-down #1 (see "Cool-Downs" on page 233), 5 minutes.

WEDNESDAY

Start: Warm-up #3 (see "Warm-Ups" on page 232), 5 minutes.

Middle: Thirty minutes of weight training, following the same format as on Monday and Friday. Some of the exercises have been replaced with others that work the same muscle group but from a different point of attack. For example, flies have been substituted for bench presses—different exercises, but both targeting the chest muscles. In other exercises, we've simply switched from barbells to dumbbells, once again in an effort to stress the muscle from a slightly different angle.

Exercise Stations: Leg press, leg curl, dumbbell fly, lat pulldown to chest, military press with dumbbells, upright row with dumbbells, tricep kickback, bicep curl with dumbbells.

Finish: Cool-down #1 (see "Cool-Downs" on page 233), 5 minutes.

Now that you know the basic programs, all you have to do is fine-tune them according to your schedule and the equipment available to you. Remember to add variety to your workouts. Trying new exercises or new combinations of exercises will keep you from going stale, both physically and mentally.

Once you've done this, you're left with two choices: Either start building a bigger, faster, healthier body, or use those 40 minutes to come up with another excuse not to exercise.

—Dan Bensimhon

Deflate Your Spare Tire

Lose your potbelly and you'll look better, feel better, have more energy and probably even live longer. Here are a dozen steps to a sleeker middle.

The potbelly spares no man. One day you wake up and you can no longer see the muscles in your abdomen. Your old pants no longer fit comfortably in the waist. Shirts that used to look great on you are starting to spread a bit between the buttons.

Middle age has caught up with your middle section. Your genes, hormones and slowing metabolism are ganging up on your gut.

It's a simple fact that if you take in more calories than you burn, the extra gets stored as fat. In men, more of that fat collects underneath the abdominal muscles than in other places—which is why some men can have rock-hard stomachs but still be thick at the equator.

Starting at about age 20, age-related changes begin to make it progressively easier for your belly to bulge. Most muscles and organs become smaller, and the body starts needing fewer calories to keep itself going. At the same time, your metabolism, or the rate at which the body burns calories, slows down.

Granted, these changes occur gradually. According to Jo-Ann Heslin, a registered dietitian and coauthor of *The Fat Attack Plan,* a man's metabolism slows only about 2 percent per decade after age 20.

"The catch is that while calorie requirements and metabolism are decreasing, most men are eating the same or more, and becoming less active," says Robert Kushner, M.D., director of the Nutrition and Weight Control Clinic at the University of Chicago. As a result, we stockpile calories. In the decade between ages 30 and 40 alone, the average man gains about six pounds.

All this is to say that a potbelly becomes more likely as you age. But it's not inevitable. The power to get rid of those extra inches is all yours. And there's good reason to do it. Lose your potbelly and you'll look better, feel better, have more energy and probably even live longer. Recent studies have linked potbellies with more serious problems such as heart disease, high blood pressure, stroke and diabetes.

Here, based on the latest research, are the best strategies for deflating that spare tire.

Exercise (But Not Necessarily Sit-Ups)

Working out reverses the processes that cause a potbelly to form by revving up the metabolism and burning calories, explains Wayne Westcott, Ph.D., YMCA national strength-training consultant. Exercise helps you take pounds off and keep them off. In a long-term weight-loss study, men who exercised gained back only half the weight of men who only dieted. Here's what you need to know.

Aerobics target the belly. Recent research shows that when men burn fat with aerobic exercises, they lose it first and fastest in the abdomen.

In a study at the University of Washington, Seattle men who took part in an intensive aerobic exercise program dropped 20 percent of the fat from their midsection in six months—almost twice the amount taken off arms and legs. Researchers dubbed this effect "preferential loss."

"Their shapes changed from round to more oblong," says researcher Robert S. Schwartz, M.D. "It was very obvious." He speculates that the more fat you have around the middle, the quicker you'll drop it with exercise.

Aerobic exercise is the cornerstone of any fat-burning plan because it does the most to fire up the metabolism. Any activity that boosts your heart rate above its resting pace for 30 minutes to an hour qualifies. Fat starts to melt away about 20 minutes into a workout, and the higher the heart rate, the more calories you'll burn. Aerobic exercise also makes your charged-up metabolism ignite calories even after you've quit your workout.

Top aerobic exercises for fat burning include cross-country skiing, stair climbing, running and biking.

Lift weights to lose waist. Weight training, long maligned as an inefficient fat burner, is now being hailed for its power to boost the benefits of aerobics. What's more, it speeds weight loss more than previously thought.

Weight training builds muscle, and muscle takes more energy to sustain itself than fat does. The more muscle you have, the higher your metabolism idles, not just after exercising, but *all* the time. "Every pound of muscle you add raises your daily calorie needs by 30 to 50 a day," says Dr. Westcott. "Over the course of an eight-week weight training program, if you gain three to five pounds of muscle—which is typical—you could be burning 250 extra calories a day just by sitting still."

This metabolic afterburn from weight training is one-third greater than that from aerobic exercise, according to a study at Oregon Health Sciences University.

The best results of all come with a one-two punch of weight training and aerobics. In a 16-week study at the University of Massachusetts, dieters doing both weights and aerobics lost more weight than dieters who did just one or the other.

Getting results from weights takes a surprisingly small commitment of time. Westcott recommends a 20-minute, thrice-weekly program requiring only one set on a typical circuit of either machines or free weights. This consists of about nine different exercises, each of which targets a major muscle group—biceps, triceps, upper back, lower back, pectorals, quadriceps, hamstrings, abdominals and shoulders. For each exercise, make the resistance heavy enough that muscles feel tired after 10 repetitions. When you can do 12 reps easily, increase the weight by 2½ to 5 pounds.

Isolate the abdominals. Can you target a bulging midsection with exercises like sit-ups and crunches? The prevailing evidence is that you cannot. Even if you were to do 300 sit-ups a day—and this has actually been tried in tests—you'd never work up enough aerobic steam to melt an ounce of flab. But evidence shows that abdominal exercises do help in a different way. Sit-ups and crunches strengthen the muscles lying atop your inner fat cavity, and that can make your belly look smaller by altering your posture, says Ellington Darden, Ph.D., director of research for Nautilus Sports/Medical Industries and author of *32 Days to a 32-Inch Waist*.

According to Dr. Darden, a heavy abdomen can tug on the spine and cause it to arch forward. That sway in the back pushes the belly out farther and can cause back strain to boot. Slow abdominal crunches help shore up the muscles that support the spine. "You're improving the whole girdle system of support in your midsection," he says.

He recommends one set of ten trunk curls and one set of ten reverse trunk curls. To do a trunk curl, lie on your back, with your arms crossed at the wrist above your chest, your knees bent and your feet flat on the floor. Slowly lift your shoulder blades, then your head, curling your chin toward your chest. Don't sit all the way up, but hold in a raised position for a count of five, then slowly lower your shoulders back to the floor. To do a reverse trunk curl, lie on your back and lift your hips toward the center of your chest. Keep your hands on the floor to help lift your buttocks off the mat.

Eat Right

For most men, diets are the weapon of choice in the attack on fat. Unfortunately, diets usually don't work in the long term, especially if you lose weight quickly. "Some can even be harmful because they create mineral imbalances, loss of fluid, constipation and diarrhea," says Dr. Kushner. Is it any wonder they make some men depressed?

Still, what you take in has a direct bearing on what you store up (and where). The good news is that you don't necessarily have to cut back on how much you eat; it's what you eat that makes the difference. "Not all calories are equivalent. It matters where they come from," says Adam Drewnowski, Ph.D., director of the human nutrition program at the University of Michigan School of Public Health. Here's the best advice on eating right.

Cut fat. Studies show it's far more important to cut fat than calories. Eating fat will make you fat. "Fat is stored more easily and doesn't burn as fast as other nutrients," Dr. Kushner says. And in men, fat calories are most likely to be stored in the abdomen. (In women, fat goes mostly to the hips, thighs and buttocks.)

Researchers at Cornell University have made the astonishing finding that cutting fat intake can make you lose weight, *no matter how much food or how many calories you take in*. In one study, all subjects ate the same kind of food, but people in a low-fat group went without mayo on their turkey sandwiches, for example, or had low-fat instead of regular yogurt. Simple measures like this allowed them to cut fat to the 25 percent of calories that experts recommend we eat. (The average man gets about 38 percent of calories from fat.) After 11 weeks, the low-fat eaters lost twice as much weight as people who ate more fat, even though there was no restriction on the total calories they consumed and the high-fat eaters limited calories to 2,000 per day.

The study's leader, David Levitsky, Ph.D., professor of nutrition

FAT GOALS

To limit fat to 25 percent of your total calorie intake, you should eat no more than the following amounts. (These figures apply to men only.)

Weight (lb.)	Calorie Intake	Fat Limit (g)
130	1,800	51
140	2,000	54
150	2,100	58
160	2,200	62
170	2,400	66
180	2,500	70
190	2,700	74
200	2,800	78

and psychology, estimates that a low-fat diet can trim 10 percent off your body weight per year.

Easy ways to cut fat from your diet are to choose low-fat or nonfat milk, cheese and yogurt; eat lean cuts of meat and trim all visible fat; and fill up on vegetables, fruits and grain products such as bread and pasta.

Load up on carbohydrates. Banish all notions that starches stick to the ribs. Carbohydrates burn fastest of all the body's energy sources and aren't easily converted into fat. When they are converted, the process itself burns calories. On top of that, carbohydrates spark the release of adrenaline, which burns still more calories. "Carbohydrates just cause the metabolic machinery in the body to turn over faster," says Dr. Kushner.

Weight-loss experts say that boosting carbohydrate intake will superheat a low-fat diet. That's because at the same time you're storing less fat by eating less of it, carbs can make your body work faster to burn the fat you have.

In one study, people placed on a fatty diet who tried to *maintain* the weight they had gained just couldn't do it when they switched to eating carbohydrates. What's more, most of the pounds they lost were fat. Body weight dropped about 3 percent on average, but body fat was cut by more than 11 percent.

Experts recommend you get about 60 percent of your calories from carbohydrates.

Tank up on water. Water's a secret weapon in the weight-loss war. Drinking more can help shed pounds in two ways.

First, it can take the edge off cravings. Often what seems like a craving for food is actually a craving for fluid, according to George L. Blackburn, M.D., Ph.D., chief of the Nutrition/Metabolism Laboratory at New England Deaconess Hospital in Boston. By drinking small sips of three or four ounces throughout the day—especially when you feel hungry—you can avert the need to indulge.

Second, if the water is ice cold, it can actually burn calories, according to Dr. Darden. "Ice-cold water is about 40°F," he says, "and it takes 226 calories of body heat to warm a gallon of it up to 98.6°." Dr. Darden recommends keeping an insulated 32-ounce bottle with a straw in it at your workplace all day. He advocates drinking four of these a day—double the usual recommendations for minimum daily fluid intake. But drinking that much icy water over a four-week period will make you drop about two pounds.

Cut Drinking and Quit Smoking

Experts say both alcohol and cigarettes cause changes in the body that make it easier for fat to pad the midsection. Here's the best advice.

Limit drinks to one a day (or thereabouts). That's what the Surgeon General recommends, and it sounds reasonable enough. But Michael Jensen, M.D., a consulting physician in nutrition, metabolism and internal medicine at the Mayo Clinic, knows this isn't how life works. One beer usually means three or four, at 100 to 200 calories per—"and that's just for the cheap stuff," he says. "That many beers, even if they're lights, could account for a third of your daily calories."

According to Dr. Jensen, there are three good reasons to cut back on alcohol if you want to lose a potbelly.

First, there are all those calories.

Second, since alcohol can't be stored the way other nutrients can, the body has to burn it off immediately. While the body's burning alcohol, it's *not* burning fat, which undermines the flab fight.

Third, beer isn't served with fruits and vegetables. "It's usually chips and dips and other things with a lot of fat and calories," Dr. Jensen says. "There's fat gain from circumstances."

One drink a day? "I wouldn't say you have to be so strict," Dr. Jensen concedes. "Make that an average. It's not the people who have an occasional three or four drinks that'll have a problem, but those who have three or four drinks *every day*." Still, he adds, "if you're concerned about a potbelly, certainly alcohol is one of the first places to cut back."

If you smoke, stop. Some people argue that cigarettes keep you thin, since the average smoker weighs less than the average nonsmoker. But study after study shows that people who smoke—even if they're lighter than people who don't—tend to have bigger bellies. Scientists speculate that smoking causes hormones to steer more fat to the midriff. Quitting detours fat from the belly, so any weight that's gained tends to gather in the legs, resulting in a more balanced-looking shape, according to researcher Robert C. Klesges, Ph.D., associate professor of psychology at Memphis State University.

What's more, Dr. Klesges and others have found in studies that quitting brings lighter-than-normal smokers only up to the weight they would have been if they'd never smoked.

Making It Work

"To increase exercise and cut down on fat sounds simple enough, but it's really pretty tough because you have to work at it every day," says Carolyn Berdanier, Ph.D., a professor of nutrition at the University of Georgia. Here's what experts suggest to make your program a success.

Be a fat-tracker. To limit fat to 25 or 30 percent of your daily calories, you'll need to monitor your intake by reading labels.

To tell how many grams of fat are in a serving, lift the number straight from the label. Tally what you eat throughout the day. The average man takes in about 2,400 calories a day. To limit fat to 25 percent of that total, he should eat no more than 67 grams of fat per day.

For menu planning, paperback books like *The Fat Counter,* which Jo-Ann Heslin co-wrote with another dietitian, Annette B. Natow, Ph.D., provide a handy fat tally for thousands of foods, including name-brand foods.

Set reasonable goals. To lose a pound of fat, you need to burn 3,500 more calories than you take in. That kind of combustion doesn't happen quickly. It's not realistic to figure on dropping 25 pounds in a month. How can you tell what is realistic? First, figure your target weight. To calculate that, give yourself 106 pounds for your first 5 feet of height. Add 6 pounds for each inch of height above that. For example, if you were 5-foot-9, you'd start with 106 pounds for the first 5 feet and add 54 (9 more inches times 6 pounds each). Your target weight would be 160. If you need to lose 20 pounds or less, you can reasonably do it in two months, says Heslin.

Make a plan. Once you decide to lose weight, wait at least two weeks before taking any action, advises Michael R. Lowe, Ph.D., associate professor of clinical psychology at Hahnemann University in Philadelphia. "Too many diets are impulsive," he says. "If you plan how you're going to diet, how you're going to work in your exercise, how you're going to eat out in different places, your commitment is likely to be stronger."

Keep a budget of daily fat, but don't forbid yourself to eat certain foods. A budget allows the flexibility to splurge on foods you crave as long as you keep the total fat count within limits. "There are no junk foods, provided you have balance and variety," says Dr. Drewnowski. "Go ahead and eat a burger. It won't kill you. Just don't have another one tomorrow."

Plot gradual changes. In the first weeks, eliminate eating in the car, for example, then banish eating in front of the TV. If you're drinking whole milk, ease into skim by first mixing whole with 2 percent. After a month, mix in 1 percent, and keep diluting until skim tastes good to you.

If you want to keep to an exercise schedule, Dr. Kushner recommends writing workouts into your calendar. "Appointments are powerful self-motivators for men," he says.

Weigh your progress. Weigh yourself every other day, advises Dr. Kushner. Men's weight doesn't fluctuate as wildly as women's, so you should see steady progress if you're sticking to your plan. Pat yourself on the back for any improvement, but don't judge yourself harshly if you suffer a setback. Even when you blow your diet a fifth of the time, that's an 80 percent success rate—good reason to keep going.

Follow these steps to banishing a potbelly, and you can retain the physique you had when you were 18 well into adulthood, according to Heslin. "There's no reason you shouldn't be able to wear the same jeans you had in your freshman year of college," she says.

—*Richard Laliberte*

It's Supposed to Be Fun, Right?

Here are myths about exercise you wish somebody had debunked when you were in junior high gym class.

When it comes to myths, there may be more about exercise than just about anything. Here are 15 you have probably heard at one time or another.

1. It's supposed to be fun. Sometimes it is, sometimes it isn't. Fun really isn't the point. The point is how good you feel *after* you've put your body through its paces.

2. Sit-ups flatten your belly. They'll tone your stomach muscles, but they won't do much to any fat that covers those muscles. You can't spot-reduce with exercise; if you could, people who chew gum a lot would all have thin faces.

3. You'll lose weight. The scale is not a good measure of how well your exercise program is working. If you lift weights, for example, you'll lose flab; but because you're losing fat tissue and replacing it with denser, heavier muscle tissue, your weight may stay the same. The important thing is, you'll look better.

4. You should work out before you eat. Only partly true. If you're more than 30 percent above your ideal weight, exercising before a meal will burn up more calories. If you're less than 30 percent overweight, exercising *after* eating burns more calories. (To avoid indigestion, however, you probably won't want to do any serious aerobic exercise too soon after eating a main meal.)

5. Machines are better than free weights. Machines may be more convenient, even safer in some cases, but you can build just as much muscle if you learn how to use barbells and dumbbells.

6. Weight lifters should eat extra protein. Most of us already have too much protein in our diets. Although exercising will use up some protein, your current intake is probably more than adequate to replenish it.

7. Morning is the best time to exercise. There's no evidence that exercising at a particular time of day is significantly more beneficial. The best time to exercise is when you most feel like exercising. If you're not a morning person, you're not going to stick with a morning workout program for long. The only caveat is that exercising too close to bedtime may make it more difficult for you to fall asleep.

8. Stretching afterward can help prevent muscle pain. Studies show that stretching after a workout has no effect on muscle soreness.

9. You have to do it for 30 minutes straight to get any benefit. A study at Stanford University showed that 10 minutes of exercise three times a day is almost as good. In any case, a little exercise every day, even if it's just a walk, is a lot better than none at all.

10. When you stop, muscle turns to fat. Hard muscles may turn into soft muscles, but they won't turn into fat. Muscle cells and fat cells are completely different and neither can ever turn into the other.

11. Sooner or later, you'll get hurt. Injuries are far from inevitable. In fact, the majority of exercisers don't get hurt. Of those that do, the most common cause is overuse. The best way to avoid injuries is to increase the intensity and duration of your exercise a little at a time.

12. After a good sweat, you'll need extra salt. You'd have to shed three quarts of sweat to lose just *half* of the 9 to 12 grams of salt the average man consumes in a day. Since it's highly unlikely you'll sweat anything close to that amount, there's no reason to add extra salt to your diet or to take salt pills after hot-weather workouts.

13. Sit-ups are best done with hands behind your neck. Not if you don't want to wreck that neck. Doing sit-ups with your hands behind your neck puts too much pressure on cervical vertebrae. Keep your hands on your chest.

14. People with high blood pressure shouldn't lift weights. People with high blood pressure, or any cardiovascular problem, should see their doctors before undertaking a strength-training exercise program, but long-term effects of weight lifting on blood pressure have failed to show any negative effects, and some have demonstrated that the exercises can *reduce* blood pressure.

15. No pain, no gain. Ignore pain, no brain. You can get very fit without feeling any serious discomfort, so don't strain when you train. If it hurts, stop it.

—Michael Lafavore

No-Pain Gain

Straight from the American College of Sports Medicine, here's a sport-by-sport guide to injury-free training.

When we were kids, we didn't have to worry much about sports injuries. Our bodies seemed to be made from some indestructible material. We could run for miles, ride our bike until the chain fell off and throw our bodies around on a baseball diamond hour after hour without suffering so much as a sore muscle. If, by some mishap, we did get hurt, we healed so quickly that it hardly mattered.

At a certain age—around the far turn of 25 or so—things started to change. Those grand impulses to slide into the cleats of the second baseman in the annual Little League father-son game got us into more trouble than they were worth. A too-long weekend run could make us hobble for a week. Just putting a little extra snap into the tennis swing or golf stroke became capable of sidelining us with back or shoulder problems.

Still, it would be a big mistake to use our body's greater susceptibility to injury as an excuse to become mere spectators. The benefits of an active lifestyle still far outweigh the potential risk of injury. It's just that we've got to be willing to acknowledge that the old bones and joints and muscles aren't quite as invulnerable as they once seemed.

To help you enjoy sports without enduring the bangs, bruises, bashes, twists and strains, *Men's Health* teamed up with selected members of the world's leading organization in sports medicine and exercise science, the American College of Sports Medicine. After spending time with some of the college's 12,000 physicians, exercise physiologists, physical therapists, nutritionists, trainers and coaches, we compiled this guide to injury-free training.

Running

Running probably exacts more of a toll on the body than any other sport. With each stride, the runner's body absorbs a force equal to two to three times his own body weight. This hammers muscles, joints and tendons. Although advances in shoe technology have helped protect runners from some of the pounding, they typically lose more training time to injuries than any other athletes.

Most common injuries: Hamstring pulls, Achilles tendinitis, shin splints (inflammation of the soft tissue in the lower leg), stress fractures in feet or lower leg.

Number of injuries treated in hospital per year: 59,525.

INJURY-FREE TRAINING TIPS

1. Walk as well as run. Especially when starting a running program, it's smart to blend in some walking. It's easier on the joints, muscles and tendons, and mile for mile, it burns almost the same number of calories as running, says cardiologist Paul Thompson, M.D., a former 2:28 marathoner.

2. Balance your body. Running primarily strengthens the muscles in the *backs* of the legs (the calves and hamstrings) while neglecting the quadriceps in the front. To balance out any strength differences, runners should do exercises such as squats and leg extensions to build up their quadriceps. Also, runners should stretch before and after running to keep their calves and hamstrings as flexible and shock-absorbent as possible.

3. Run in running shoes; walk in walking shoes. "Many runners live in their running shoes, and this is asking for injury," says Dr. Thompson. Running shoes have very little heel, and they tend to leave the Achilles tendon unsupported when you walk. Walking shoes don't offer enough cushioning for a run.

4. Up your mileage gradually. Trying to do too much too soon is probably the surest way to get hurt. A good rule of thumb is never to increase your weekly mileage by more than 10 percent.

5. Run on soft surfaces. Choose dirt or grass-covered trails over concrete or asphalt.

Swimming

More Americans participate in swimming than any other sport, and that makes doctors very happy. Unlike dry-land athletes, swimmers don't have to support their own weight, so their bodies are spared the jarring forces that so often cause injuries. When swimmers do hurt themselves, the injuries are usually from overuse or improper form.

Most common injuries: Swimmer's shoulder (rotator-cuff strains or tears), elbow tendinitis, knee pain.

Number of injuries treated in hospital per year: 33,407.

INJURY-FREE TRAINING TIPS

1. Get your strokes down. Improper stroke techniques are the cause of many swimming injuries, says Rick Sharp, Ph.D., editor of the *Journal of Swimming Research*. Have a knowledgeable swimmer or coach analyze your stroke to correct any mechanical problems.

2. Mix it up. Doing a variety of strokes during your swim workout will decrease your chances of suffering an overuse injury.

3. Keep things rolling. Shoulder injuries are more common in freestyle swimmers who have a flat stroke than in those who roll their shoulders into the water.

4. Turn up the volume slowly. Like other endurance athletes, swimmers tend to get injured when they try to do too much too soon. Never increase the amount of swimming you do in a single workout or training week by more than 10 percent.

Racquetball

Locked in a small room with one or more racket-swinging opponents and a hard rubber ball cruising at 80 to 100 miles an hour, racquetball players are at considerable risk for eye injury. But also common are lacerations and bruises from head-on collisions with walls and opponents; muscle pulls and strains from overly vigorous serves and returns; and joint and ligament sprains and tears from the constant stop-start action.

Most common injuries: Elbow and wrist tendinitis, ankle sprains, hamstring pulls, eye injuries, lacerations.

Number of injuries treated in hospital per year: 12,944.

INJURY-FREE TRAINING TIPS

1. Learn your strokes. As with any racket sport, improper stroke mechanics are the surest path to overuse injuries like elbow or wrist tendinitis, says Garron Weiker, M.D., administrative director of the Section of Sports Medicine at the Cleveland Clinic Foundation. Even if you've been playing for several years, sign up for a session with a teaching pro who can evaluate your strokes and tell you if you need to make any changes.

2. Get a good racket. A high-quality racket with a comfortable grip can help reduce tendinitis-producing vibration and shock. (Whether you choose aluminum or graphite makes little difference from an injury standpoint as long as the racket is well made, notes Dr. Weiker.)

3. Watch your eyes. Eye protection is a must for all racquetball players. "Although many players wear open (i.e., lensless) goggles, these do not give full protection since a speeding racquetball can bulge through the opening," says Dr. Weiker. Wraparound goggles with solid polycarbonate lenses are your best bet.

4. Get court shoes. Rubber-soled racquetball shoes are the best for the game, but in a pinch, a tennis, basketball or cross-training shoe will give you the heel support and cushioning you need to avoid injury.

Tennis

Nearly half of all tennis players suffer from tennis elbow (pain usually caused by tendinitis) at least once. The problem stems from repeatedly making strokes that require wrist action and rotation of the forearm. Tennis players also suffer from lower back and shoulder injuries resulting from vigorous serves and overheads. Tears and sprains in the leg muscles are also common because of the stop-start motion required for the game.

Most common injuries: Shoulder and elbow tendinitis, knee tendinitis and cartilage damage, back strains, rotator-cuff tears.

Number of injuries treated in hospital per year: 34,674.

INJURY-FREE TRAINING TIPS

1. Muscle up. Contrary to common belief, frequent tennis playing actually *weakens* the shoulder muscles by stretching and fatiguing the tissues there, says Robert Nirschl, M.D., medical director and orthopedic consultant at the Virginia Sports Medicine Institute in Arlington. To reduce their risk of shoulder injury, all tennis players need to perform strengthening exercises targeting their arms and shoulders. Good exercises include wrist curls, shoulder shrugs and shoulder rolls.

2. Get good form. "Improper technique can cause a whole host of injuries," says Dr. Nirschl. Even if you've been playing for years, the odds are that your stroke mechanics could use some fine-tuning. Taking a lesson or two every month will help you develop and maintain proper form.

3. Stretch your back before you play. For a simple stretch, lie on your back, grasp one leg underneath the knee with both hands and gently pull it toward your chest, then repeat with the other leg.

4. Go graphite. Graphite rackets are lightweight and strong, a perfect combination for damping injury-producing vibration.

5. Don't be so tense. String the racket at the lowest tension possible. High string tensions provide good control over the ball but pass along more vibration to the arm.

6. Get tennis shoes. Tennis shoes are specifically designed to give you the right traction, cushioning and heel support to keep your feet and lower legs healthy after hours on the court. In a pinch, cross-training shoes will do the trick, although by using them you may sacrifice some traction and support.

Basketball/Volleyball

With all their quick starts, sudden stops and sky-high leaps, these two sports are among the most exciting around. But all this excitement does have its price, especially for the unprepared body.

First, there's the tremendous amount of lateral force both place on ankles and knees. Then there's the bone- and joint-jarring jumping, which sends injurious shock waves throughout the body. All this adds up to a simple, undeniable conclusion: Basketball and volleyball players who want to stay healthy need to work extra hard between games to stay in shape.

Most common injuries: Ankle sprains, knee cartilage or ligament strains and tears, knee or Achilles tendinitis, assorted muscle strains.

Number of injuries treated in hospital per year: basketball, 465,616; volleyball, 87,023.

INJURY-FREE TRAINING TIPS

1. Get the right shoes. Shoes designed specifically for basketball or volleyball provide the support, cushioning and traction needed to play the game injury-free, says Bert Mandelbaum, M.D., team physician at Pepperdine University in California. Wear high-tops, especially if you have weak ankles. Doing so can greatly reduce the chance of reinjuring a previously sprained or strained ankle.

2. Prepare your body. The constant jumping and stop-start motion of basketball and volleyball can easily injure muscles that aren't trained to deal with these motions. Agility drills (doing short bursts of running from side to side) can help prepare an athlete's body to absorb these tremendous forces, says Peter Bruno, M.D., internist for the New York Rangers and Knicks.

3. Protect your eyes for basketball. Though it's not officially a contact sport, elbows and hands do tend to find their way into your eyes. To best protect your visual assets without reducing your vision, use wraparound polycarbonate lenses. The lenses are lightweight and unbreakable, and they provide protection from all possible angles.

4. Get padded for volleyball. If you're one of those players who'll do anything to put themselves between the ball and the floor, wear neoprene elbow pads and kneepads.

Baseball

Anyone who repeatedly throws a ball at high speeds is at risk of damaging his rotator cuff, the group of muscles and tendons that surround the shoulder joint. To protect this sensitive area, it's essential to work on upper-body strength and flexibility. And since baseball itself does little to improve overall fitness, it is extremely important for base-ball players to maintain their own independent conditioning program.

Most common injuries: Elbow or shoulder tendinitis, rotator-cuff tears, bruises and scrapes.

Number of injuries treated in hospital per year: 280,652.

INJURY-FREE TRAINING TIPS

1. Build gradually. Throwing too much or too hard at the begin-ning of the season is a sure way to injure untrained muscles, says Dennis Wilson, Ed.D., head of the Department of Health and Human Performance at Auburn University in Alabama.

2. Muscle up. Although it's impossible to *strengthen* the rotator cuff itself with a single exercise, you can protect it by doing weight-lifting exercises to build the shoulder and upper back muscles. Lateral raises, rowing-type exercises and lat pulldowns are all great exercises for baseball players.

3. Warm up. Although baseball requires explosive bursts of activity, the game itself provides little opportunity for a player to warm his mus-cles. Thus it's necessary to make time for a pregame warm-up consisting of some short jogs and stretches for the shoulders, back and legs.

4. Get spiked. Molded-plastic cleats are best for baseball since they provide more traction than running or court shoes and they're less dangerous than metal spikes.

Cycling

Even though cycling doesn't involve the pounding common to many sports, bike riders suffer more injuries than any other group of athletes. Falls do most of the damage, but the constant pedaling can also cause injury by repeatedly stressing the same muscles. Finally, the prolonged hunched-over position puts cyclists at risk for back pain.

Most common injuries: Knee tendinitis, low back muscle strain, cuts and scrapes.

Number of injuries treated in hospital per year: 580,119.

INJURY-FREE TRAINING TIPS

1. Put a lid on. The majority of cycling injuries are the result of crashes or falls. A recent study found that one life could be saved every day in the United States if all cyclists were to wear helmets.

2. Get a good fit. Many cyclists experience chronic back and knee pain from improper positioning on their bikes, says Jim Hagberg, Ph.D., exercise physiologist at the University of Maryland. To get a proper fit, have an experienced rider or bike mechanic check the position of your saddle, handlebars and cleats.

3. Train your stomach. Building strong abdominal muscles can give your back the support it needs while you're cycling. Do abdominal-strengthening exercises like crunches two or three times a week to ward off back pain.

4. Spin, don't strain. Although using bigger, higher gears can make you go faster, it can also make you more susceptible to muscle strains and other overuse injuries. "Using lower gears and a faster pedal stroke is not only easier on the body, it's also more efficient," says Dr. Hagberg.

5. Wear proper cycling shoes. Firm-soled cycling shoes make pedaling more efficient and help reduce strain on your feet.

6. Protect your eyes. Sunglasses not only reduce fatigue from the sun's glare but also keep flying debris and insects out of your eyes. When shopping for glasses, look for ones with polycarbonate lenses that are labeled "special purpose." The polycarbonate material prevents shattering, while the special-purpose label ensures maximum protection from the sun's ultraviolet rays.

Bowling

Once-a-week bowlers run the risk of straining underdeveloped muscles from hefting those 16-pound balls. And those who bowl daily are at risk for overuse injuries. Whether you're an avid bowler or gutter-ball specialist, it pays to prepare for the demands the sport places on your body.

Most common injuries: Elbow tendinitis, wrist tendinitis, knee, back and shoulder strains, blisters.

Number of injuries treated in hospital per year: 22,515.

INJURY-FREE TRAINING TIPS

1. Watch that hook. Trying to put too much spin on the ball is one of the major causes of bowling injuries. If you decide you need to develop a spin delivery, switch to a lighter ball until you get the form down.

2. Adjust your form to your physique. If you have a bad back, don't bend at the back as much when you throw; instead, bend your knees to get low to the ground for your delivery. If you've had a knee injury, bend more at the back and keep your knees a bit straighter for your delivery.

3. Don't whip it. A smooth delivery that allows you to put your entire body behind the ball is the most effective, and safest, way to generate ball speed. Whipping or jerking the ball from your shoulder greatly increases your risk of injury—and gutter balls.

4. Don't rent shoes. Even if you only bowl once a month, it's both fiscally and physically wise to buy your own shoes. Not only will they look better, they'll also give you the proper fit and traction you need to ward off injuries.

Golf

Golfers are susceptible to back injuries. With every swing of the club, a golfer bends forward, rotates at the hips and then follows through with as much force and speed as he can muster. All this puts tremendous strain on both the lower and upper back muscles.

Most common injuries: Low back strains, shoulder strains, shoulder, wrist and elbow tendinitis.

Number of injuries treated in hospital per year: 35,218.

INJURY-FREE TRAINING TIPS

1. Stay loose. Since golf involves a great deal of rotation at the shoulders and hips, keeping these areas flexible is the most important thing you can do to prevent injuries, says Lewis Yocum, M.D., assistant medical director for the Professional Golfers' Association of America. For a simple shoulder stretch, raise your right arm straight above your head, then bend it at the elbow so your right hand falls behind your neck. With your left hand, gently pull your right elbow. Stop when you feel a gentle stretch in your right shoulder and hold for five seconds. Repeat with the other arm. To stretch your back and hips, stand with your feet flat on the floor, shoulder-width apart. While holding a golf club behind your neck, twist your upper body gently from side to side without moving your feet.

2. Muscle up. Strengthening your back and abdominal muscles will also decrease your chance of golf injuries. The best exercises for golf involve rotational motion. Try diagonal sit-ups (where you alternately bring your right elbow to your left knee and left elbow to your right knee).

3. Use the proper shoes. As in any other sport, having the right shoes for golf is vital. You really do need those little spikes to hold your feet in place as you make the backswing. As for the tassels, well, it's your call.

4. Take a lesson. Improper form greatly increases your risk of injury. To keep yourself from developing any bad habits in your game, take a few lessons from a teaching pro at your local golf course. Even if you've got a five handicap, it's a good idea to have a pro analyze your stroke at least once a season.

5. Don't whack it. A fluid stroke that generates a lot of club speed is the key to driving a golf ball far down the fairway. "Trying to muscle a ball off the tee will only get you injured," says Dr. Yocum. Also, when practicing your drive, hit off a soft surface such as grass. Constantly hitting off a hard plastic mat transfers a great deal of shock to your lower arm and can cause tendinitis.

6. Squat, don't bend. There's a lot of reaching to place or pick up balls in this game. Bending over at the waist can place a great deal of strain on your lower back. Remember to bend your knees before leaning forward.

—Dan Bensimhon

Damage Control

Oooow! Sometimes, despite all precautions, sports injuries happen. Here's what to do when you're hurting.

Playing sports is supposed to be fun. It's not supposed to hurt. If it's more pain than pleasure, you're definitely doing something wrong. Usually such twinges, strains, muscle pulls and cramps are your body's way of telling you that you've been pushing too hard. Pay attention.

Probably the most common of all exercise pains is *muscle soreness,* dull pain that usually shows up within a day of strenuous exercise. There's no reason to stop exercising because of a minor ache, but go easy for a day or two. Gentle stretching and a massage can also help reduce the stiffness associated with muscle aches. The ache should disappear completely within 72 hours. If it doesn't, see a doctor.

Muscle cramps can range from a mildly painful lockup of a muscle group to an agonizing stabbing feeling. What's happening is a lot like what it *feels* is happening: Your muscle has contracted and won't release. It's usually caused by muscle fatigue, dehydration or chemical imbalance. If you get a cramp while exercising, stop or slow down until the pain goes away. (It usually will in a minute or two.) Some find that stretching or rubbing the muscle helps speed the recovery process.

Muscle strains and pulls range from mild overstretching to an actual tear. Sometimes the first signal is a twinge during a workout; other times the pain is sudden and searing. In the first case go easy and see if the pain dissipates. If not, or if the pain is severe, stop exercising and treat the injury with R.I.C.E. (see "R.I.C.E to the Rescue" on page 257). Consult a doctor if pain hasn't begun to ease within 48 hours. A strain may take several weeks to heal.

Here, from the American College of Sports Medicine, are some more specific tips on dealing with sports injuries.

Foot

Symptoms: Sharp pain directly over one of the bones in the foot, usually accompanied by slight swelling. Pain increases during exercise or when standing for long periods.

Probable injury: Stress fracture of one of the small bones in the foot, often caused by the repetitive pounding of running.

Treatment: Stop activity. See a physician.

Prevention: Wear shoes with good cushioning. Run on softer surfaces such as grass or an indoor track. Increase training gradually.

Symptoms: Pain and tenderness that begin in the heel and radiate into the midsection of the foot. Pain lessens during activity but returns intensely an hour or so after stopping.

255

Probable injury: Plantar fasciitis, an inflammation of the connective tissue that runs from the heel bone to the base of the toes and supports the bottom of the foot.

Treatment: Rest. Ice. Over-the-counter pain relievers (before taking any medication, check with your physician on dosage, indications and side effects). Orthotics to reduce overpronation and remove stress from the fascia.

Prevention: Wear shoes with good arch support and cushioning. Use orthotics to prevent overpronation. Keep fascia flexible and strong by scrunching up a towel with your toes.

Ankle

Symptoms: Pain and swelling, usually on outside of ankle after trauma. Commonly accompanied by bruising.

Probable injury: Ankle sprain, a stretching or tearing of ankle ligaments. Damage ranges from mild overstretching to complete rupture.

Treatment: R.I.C.E. If pain persists or worsens over 48 hours, see a doctor.

Prevention: Keep ankles flexible and strong with the following exercise: Wrap a towel around the ball of your foot and extend your ankle as you pull back on the towel to provide resistance. Wear a brace or high-top sneakers to support previously injured ankles. Run on even surfaces.

Lower Leg

Symptoms: Burning pain on the back of the leg near the heel. Pain lessens with activity but returns soon after stopping. May be accompanied by swelling and redness.

Probable injury: Achilles tendinitis, an inflammation in the tendon that connects the calf muscle to the heel bone.

Treatment: Rest. Ice. Over-the-counter pain relievers. Stretch tendon gently when pain is gone by standing 18 inches from a wall and leaning into the wall while keeping feet flat on floor. Place heel lift in shoe to decrease stretch of Achilles and help prevent reinjury.

Prevention: Wear shoes with adequate heel support and cushioning. Stretch regularly. Increase training gradually.

R.I.C.E. TO THE RESCUE

When it comes to treating injuries like sprains, pulls and tears, R.I.C.E. is the gold standard among sports-medicine professionals. This treatment helps to reduce the damage and swelling caused by an injury and can significantly speed healing.

Rest. Stop exercising—immediately. Decrease weight on the injured area (or eliminate it altogether) to prevent any further damage.

Ice. Apply ice wrapped in a towel or plastic bag to the injured spot for 10 to 20 minutes three to four times a day until acute injury subsides.

Compress. Apply pressure to the area by wrapping it in a snug (but not tight) elastic bandage.

Elevate. Lift the injured limb 12 to 18 inches and rest it on a pillow or cushion. This will reduce swelling.

Symptoms: Sharp pain in the front or back of the lower leg that typically lessens with activity but returns intensely soon after stopping. In some cases, pain may be severe during exercise as well.

Probable injury: Shin splints, an inflammation of the soft tissues in the lower leg.

Treatment: Rest. Ice. Over-the-counter pain relievers.

Prevention: Strengthen lower leg by performing exercises such as heel raises and toe raises. Increase flexibility with calf stretches. Wear shoes with good cushioning. Increase training gradually. Run on soft surfaces.

Knee

Symptoms: Deep ache or pain underneath the knee. Discomfort increases during activity, when bending or straightening knee or when direct pressure is applied. May swell or grind.

Probable injury: Chondromalacia patellae ("runner's knee"), a wearing away of the back side of the kneecap and the cartilage that cushions it.

Treatment: Rest until pain subsides (may take several weeks). Over-the-counter pain relievers. If pain persists or grinding is present, see a doctor.

Prevention: Strengthen quadriceps to better support the knee by doing leg extensions. Stretch quadriceps and hamstrings. Wear well-cushioned shoes. Have running stride analyzed to correct biomechanical flaws.

Symptoms: Intense pain along joint line that intensifies with activity. Can be accompanied by swelling or locking of joint.

Probable injury: Strain or tear of knee cartilage or ligament.

Treatment: R.I.C.E. Over-the-counter pain relievers. If pain or swelling is very severe or persists for more than 72 hours, see a doctor.

Prevention: Some injury due to trauma may be unavoidable. But you can reduce risk. Strengthen quadriceps. Keep knee flexible with stretching exercises. Wear an elastic knee brace if you have prior knee injury.

Upper Leg

Symptoms: Sharp pain on back of leg above knee can radiate to buttocks. Typically intensifies with exercise.

Probable injury: Strain or tear in hamstring muscle or the tendons that run along the back of the upper leg. (Also possible back injury. See "Back" below.)

Treatment: Rest. Ice. Switch to heat afterward, but only if it reduces pain more effectively. Gentle stretching when pain subsides. A good stretch: Lie on your back with your legs up against a wall. Slowly slide buttocks toward wall until you feel a gentle tug at the back of your legs.

Prevention: Always warm up and stretch hamstrings before exercising. Strengthen hamstring muscles and quadriceps to remove any strength imbalances. Good hamstring exercise: leg curl on an exercise machine.

Groin

Symptoms: Sharp pain in groin area that may radiate to upper thigh or lower abdomen. Typically intensifies with exercise or stretching.

Probable injury: Groin pull, a strain or partial tear in the muscles or tendons in the upper leg and lower abdomen.

Treatment: Rest. Ice. Switch to heat after first 24 hours if it helps relieve pain. Resume training gradually, as complete recovery may take up to several weeks.

Prevention: Warm up before doing any sprinting or vigorous exercise. Keep the muscles of the upper, inner thighs strong and flexible. At-home method: Wearing light ankle weights, lie on your side, lift one leg and return slowly. Do ten repetitions. Repeat with other leg.

Back

Symptoms: Ache or pain in lower back that typically subsides during exercise but can return with a vengeance afterward. Usually accompanied by stiffness. In severe cases it is difficult to sit or stand.

Probable injury: Strain in muscles of lower back. Possible herniated disk.

Treatment: Rest. Ice. Switch to heat afterward if it reduces pain better. Gentle stretching when pain subsides. See a doctor if pain intensifies over several days, radiates to buttocks or legs or causes numbness or tingling.

Prevention: Increase flexibility of back muscles by stretching daily. Strengthen abdominal muscles to support the spine. Try stomach crunches: Lie on your back with knees bent and curl your chin to your chest so your shoulders come a couple of inches off the ground. Always avoid quick, twisting motions or heavy lifting.

Shoulder

Symptoms: Dull ache or pain typically felt in the outer part of the shoulder that may radiate into the upper arm. Pain usually becomes worse with exercise. May be accompanied by swelling or redness.

Probable injury: Tendinitis (inflammation of the shoulder tendons) or bursitis (inflammation of the tiny shock-absorbing sacs inside the shoulder joint).

Treatment: Rest. Ice. Over-the-counter pain relievers. Gentle stretching when pain subsides. For a shoulder stretch, grab your right elbow with your left hand and gently pull it across your chest. Repeat with other arm.

Prevention: Strengthen shoulder muscles with rowing exercises. Increase shoulder flexibility through stretching. Always warm up before vigorous exercise.

Elbow

Symptoms: Sharp pain on outside of elbow that may radiate down forearm. Pain usually intensifies with exercise.

Probable injury: Tennis elbow, tendinitis in the elbow and surrounding portion of forearm.

Treatment: Rest. Ice. Over-the-counter pain relievers. If you continue to play, use a splint or brace to restrict wrist movement.

Prevention: Learn proper technique for your sport. Use proper equipment for your size and ability. Strengthen and stretch forearm muscles with wrist curls.

—Dan Bensimhon

Time Bandit

Is your schedule already crammed with too much work? Here are some ideas on how to fit fitness into your day.

Ron Hill remembers the day as if the past 21 years had been but a blink: the time (not much), the place (a ramshackle train platform in Stuttgart, West Germany), the reason (a hurried trip to the 1969 European track championships in Budapest).

Five years earlier, after running poorly in the Tokyo Olympics, the Englishman had vowed never again to waver in his training. And he stuck to it; not a day passed without a run. Now, though, Hill's day was slipping away, the opportunity for laps with it. At Stuttgart, he did what had to be done. He hopped off the car and did a half mile near the station, capping his effort with a final sprint to catch the departing train.

"If you want to exercise you'll find the time. It's really no different than finding the time to shave or eat," reasons Hill, who currently fits two daily runs into a hectic schedule as owner of a sportswear business in Cheshire, England. "If you want to do it, you'll do it."

The benefits of exercise have been breathlessly documented by everyone from cardiologists to reformed rock stars, every newly minted expert urging us to walk, run, heft and gyrate. Unfortunately, this advice is often effectively smothered by a more pertinent question: Where's the time?

First, realize that a little effort goes a long way. "If all you want to do is enjoy a long, healthy life, it doesn't take that much activity at all," says Kenneth Cooper, M.D., head of the Dallas-based Institute for Aerobics Research. On the other hand, there's Dr. Cooper's coronary corollary: "The majority of the patients I take care of, the ones that don't have time for fitness," he says, "find the time after that first heart attack. Time is really just an excuse."

No Excuses

Finding time, say experienced exercisers, is a matter of discipline and organization. Brent Knudsen, a 34-year-old triathlete and vice-president of marketing for a Fortune 500 company, trains every day, despite the demands of a 55-hour workweek. His regimen includes bicycling, running and a lunchtime swim at a health club.

What he does, though, isn't as important as how he does it. He maps out a schedule at the beginning of each month and then sticks to it as best he can. Planning a month in advance, Knudsen admits, is "probably a little extreme," but a schedule, even an elastic one, is essential to any successful exercise program.

"You have to schedule exercise into your day just like you'd schedule in a business meeting and, just like a business meeting, make it a priority," says Knudsen, who lives in La Jolla, California. "A lot of times work will pile up, and by noon I'll be thinking, 'I just can't swim today.'

"I just have to tell myself that I'm going to go, that I'm going to discipline myself and do it. The key is to schedule it and then commit to it."

When to fit in exercise is a matter of personal preference and, at times, no small degree of innovation. California triathlete Mike Pigg once killed time on a boat trip by carting along a stationary bike, lashing it to the deck, mounting up and spinning away. (This is a guy who apparently believes idle legs are the devil's workout; Pigg will talk to you while standing on one leg. "Builds up your knee and ankle," he explains.)

Blow Off Your Day

Less attention-grabbing, maybe a bit more productive, Knudsen cycles nightly on a stationary bike while reading reports he set aside during the day. Hill, who gets a daily run in before breakfast, recommends working out early, as fewer conflicts are apt to pop up at 6:00 A.M. Others swear by the regenerative boost of a noon sweat. Exercising later in the day can help you blow off steam from work.

"When I get to 4:00 in the afternoon I've just about had it with this place," says Tom Ponte, 45, an administrator with Aetna Life and Casualty in Hartford, Connecticut. Lately, he's been getting in at 8:00 A.M. so he can leave an hour early and put in 20 minutes to an hour at the company's fitness center.

The point is that when you choose to exercise is not as important as settling into a routine. "Once you establish a pattern you're less likely to miss a workout," explains Ponte, who has watched throngs of coworkers start a fitness program, miss a day or two, and then let everything fall by the wayside.

Fitness often seems like something you have to grab in big bunches. The truth is, in certain respects, exercise is really no different than sex or income tax refunds. "A little bit is better than nothing," says Hill. "If all you have is 20 minutes to spare, get out there and use that 20 minutes. It's always worth the effort."

When it comes to finding time, a regular exercise program can have a beneficial backlash. "Generally as people become more physically fit, they may find that they need less sleep," says Lisa Mueller, health promotion manager for Minneapolis-based Honeywell. "You may find yourself with more hours in the day to fit in exercise."

Try Push-Ups

Whenever you're feeling time-crimped, Aetna exercise physiologist Doug Barber recommends one exercise above all others: push-ups. These gym class stalwarts, combined with chair dips and crunches, make for a threesome that will work most of the major muscle groups of the upper body. Do 15 to 20 minutes of these strength exercises three times a week, along with about 20 minutes of cardiovascular work thrice weekly (walking, running, bicycling, etc.), and you'll get all the exercise you need, Barber says.

Other experts emphasize cross-training: choosing a number of exercises, then mixing them up as often as possible. This may seem straightforward, but a surprising number of people home in on one exercise, then butt heads with it until their brains turn to mush. As Doug Gambrel, an exercise physiologist for GTE in Stamford, Connecticut, says, "A variety of activities not only works muscles throughout the whole body but also keeps you fresh."

Variety, Gambrel points out, also allows for adaptability, especially important to the traveler trying to hack out an exercise program on unfamiliar, and sometimes unfriendly, turf. Running can take on a real sense of urgency in certain urban areas, but if you also lift weights or swim, it's easier to revise your schedule. Such revisions are made simpler still by the many hotels and handful of airports that offer in-house health facilities. Even if those facilities aren't available, there are still no excuses.

"If you make the commitment, you can get it done," says Tom Sullivan, a 42-year-old Hollywood actor, producer and lecturer who spent 220 days on the road last year and rarely missed a workout—an accomplishment all the more impressive considering he is blind.

Sullivan brings an elastic exercise band and a jump rope everywhere, but he actually starts each day by rolling out of bed and right to the floor for a short bout of calisthenics. It's a routine he has adopted out of respect for the realities of travel. "I don't care how disciplined you are, when you check into that hotel after a full day of traveling, exercise isn't at the top of your agenda. If you don't do it in the morning, you won't do it."

He also makes an attempt to eat lightly on the road, as does South African golf great Gary Player, who is a regimented exerciser. "Eating properly on the road is a great way to stay in shape," Player says. He makes a special effort to steer clear of fatty foods, no easy feat on the opulent Professional Golfers' Association tour.

Making Time Is Worth the Time

Let's face it, finding time for exercise can be a headache. And exercise itself is rarely the fuzzy buzz of orgiastic endorphins we would like it to be. So why not snap off the alarm and doze, forget the evening run and plow into the cheese dip?

That question is best answered by Walt Stack, who has rarely done either. As a laborer in San Francisco, Stack's day began at 2:40 in the morning, allowing him time to swim, bike and run before reporting to work at 7:30. Now that he is retired, his daily program, with minor alterations, consists of 14 miles of bicycling, 17 miles of running back and forth across the Golden Gate Bridge and a quarter-mile swim in the bay.

Stack tells you what you probably already know.

"The difficult things in this world are solved through motivation," says Stack, who is 83. "No matter how tired you are, no matter how busy you are, if you're determined, you can always make the time. It's completely up to you."

—*Ken McAlpine*

Step Up in Life

There must be a reason stair-climbing machines continue to climb in popularity. Here it is: You can burn 2,000 calories in three 30-minute workouts a week.

Stair-climbing machines have ascended in popularity so quickly that even though they've only been widely available for about a year, they already rank as the most-used type of exercise equipment in U.S. health clubs. Their fast rise to fame is probably due to the fast results they bring: Three 30-minute workouts a week on a "stepper" can burn up *2,000* calories. That regimen—along with cutting out one tablespoon of butter a day and trading in a daily glass of whole milk for a glass of low-fat—could help you shed a pound a week.

Moving your legs up and down on the steps pits muscles against resistance created by pistons, shock absorbers, or some other sort of adjustable mechanical linkage. The machines are great for developing the calves, thighs and buttocks, and you get a good cardiovascular workout in the bargain. Models with movable handles also help condition your upper body.

Stepping is low-impact exercise compared with running. And the risk of muscle strain is much less than in weight training, says Patrick Netter, a Los Angeles fitness consultant and author of the book *High-Tech Fitness:* "Stepping is less explosive, more controlled and rhythmical." It's also a good move for guys who get saddle soreness or lower back pain from riding a stationary bike, says Netter.

You can buy low-end models for less than $200 or pay ten times that for a top-of-the-line climber. Most machines are computerized. Very sophisticated units let you program different warm-up, workout and cool-down sessions.

You may not need a $2,000 climber, but don't aim too low, warns Netter: "Low-end steppers are like low-end stationary bikes: They're unstable and noisy." He also likes models with at least some electronics. "Computerization provides instantaneous feedback, which can help motivate you," Netter says.

Among Netter's picks is the midpriced Precor 7.4: "It's almost as smooth as a $2,500 unit and has some of the same electronics, but costs under $900." Whatever type you use, follow these steps for maximum results.

• Hold the handrails for balance only. The weight's got to be on your legs to guarantee the maximum burn. If you have to hang on to keep the pace, you're going too fast.

• Make sure your knees move forward, staying over your toes. If you place your foot ahead of your knee and then try to lift up on that foot, your knee could get strained. Stair climbing isn't hazardous to knees when done properly. However, if you have an existing knee injury, you probably should stay off climbers and get your exercise by walking. Check with your doctor.

• On programmable models, customize your workout time. You aren't stuck with the workout the computer has programmed (usually 15 minutes). If you want to go to 20 minutes, check your owner's manual or ask your health club trainer for programming instructions.

• Be specific. To tone buttocks muscles, take higher steps, letting the machine carry your foot farther down. To work the abdominals, take shorter steps, keeping your feet a little forward of your upper torso.

• Put the machine in a cool spot in your home. A room comfortable for couch reclining may seem like a sauna while you're step inclining. And despite the obvious jokes about "Stairway to Heaven," rock music isn't the best accompaniment to your workout. The beat is too dominant, which can throw off your pacing. Show tunes or classical music are better choices.

If you buy a stair climber, will you use it or will it become another expensive rack to throw your clothes on when you get home from work? Netter says despite the intensity of the exercise, there's a high adherence to stair climbing compared with rowing and riding stationary bikes. "It could be the rhythmic nature of the workout," he says. "You go into almost a meditative state."

—*Gloria McVeigh*

PART 10

Taking Care of Business

Breaking Free

How to jump-start a stalled career. Climbing the corporate ladder is tougher than ever—you need an edge.

He's 41; his boss is 33. He hasn't had a promotion in six years, and he's beginning not to care anymore whether he's dressed for success—or even whether his socks match. Meet a man standing on a plateau, joined by a growing number of disillusioned middle managers whose careers seem to have leveled off well short of the executive suite.

Once upon a time, and not that long ago, the path to corporate success was as automatic as an escalator. You got a good education, started with a good company, and unless you had an affair with the boss's wife, you could expect to be promoted roughly every 12 to 18 months.

But no longer. Some corporate climbs are now about as negotiable as the north face of Everest, and the reason is simple: Not only do the paths to the summit have fewer handholds, but also an unprecedented number of hands are reaching for them. Pressured to increase efficiency and profits in an ever-toughening global market, many companies started trimming their managerial ranks back in the early 1980s, and the cuts continue today. Accompanying those cuts has been a record number of 30- to 45-year-old baby boomers hitting what they thought would be their corporate stride. The result: a new upward immobility dubbed the "plateau effect"—a log-jam of well-qualified would-be CEOs finding themselves stuck in the middle levels.

Things are expected to get worse before they get better. Managerial staffs are expected to be shaved by another two-thirds by the year 2000. What's a would-be VIP looking for his fair share of the good life to do?

Men's Health posed that question to some experts who keep their fingers on the pulse of such affairs, and it seems there may be some good answers after all for men whose careers have stalled.

Seek the Jagged Path

"There's a lot of talk about this plateau effect, and a lot of griping, but only because it's being looked at in the wrong way," says Greenville, South Carolina, career counselor Al Hafer. "There's more to life and more to a career than following an uninterrupted path upward."

Hafer coped with a plateau of his own as a 40-year-old middle manager at G.E. several years back. So he began studying for his master's degree in counseling—planning to use it to develop new capabilities at work. His job expanded, but he saw greater potential in working for himself. He took early retirement and started his own business in career counseling—simultaneously going for an Ed.D. Now he advises people on the very problem he solved. "I'm my own boss, and I feel I'm doing something that's important," he says. "I'm not going to say it was easy for all the years I had to attend classes at night while also working, but hard work was never what I was afraid of."

Nor was hard work the fear of Richard Geissler, who at the age of 32 found a way around the ceiling he hit in his career as a newspaper reporter. When he was bypassed for a position as city editor in favor of a 30-year-old newcomer, he asked to be transferred to his paper's state capital bureau and, before long, joined a senator's staff in Washington. At age 50, he's now a worldwide speaker for a major trade organization and feels that reaching a plateau may have been the best thing that ever happened to him: "It got my juices going. It made me look hard at my options. It got me thinking more creatively than I ever would have if I had stayed where I was."

It's not always a question of whether you should stay or leave, points out Henry de Montebello, 44, of the executive search firm Russell Reynolds Associates. Staying with your company but moving laterally can broaden your abilities, offer new challenges and even help prepare you in the event a higher position should open up. "The executives who thrive in the future will be well rounded," says de Montebello. "You can't be a specialist at senior levels anymore; you have to be a generalist—someone who can see the big picture, a 'people person' who knows how to motivate."

David Hogberg, formerly of Quaker Oats, can vouch for that. By stepping laterally from manufacturing to product development and then to a post as a marketing manager, he not only avoided a plateau, he also gained the broad base of experience he would eventually need to win a top post. "My lateral moves were deliberate and they worked," he boasts at the relatively ripe age of 37. Today he's senior product manager at Con Agra.

Lateral mobility may indeed be the plateau antidote for many, experts say, especially if financial circumstances preclude a more entrepreneurial approach. Many large companies now are actually encouraging it, using internal job-posting systems as a way of helping employees out of the plateau trap.

All Careers Are Not Created Equally

Some careers are more likely to stall than others. This advice may be a bit late if you've already started your boardroom climb, but experts warn you to beware of positions in purchasing, personnel or data processing. The market for talent in these fields will stay level or shrink in the coming years, according to a business publication. Also steer clear of public relations (there's a big move toward doing corporate image work in-house), and avoid anything associated with the management of a company's real estate portfolio (especially while real estate remains soft). Accountants get regular pay raises but tend not to rise much in rank, and managers of all kinds who work overseas tend to forfeit the inside track to their brethren who stay close to the home office.

Other jobs are relatively immune to the plateau effect—in particular, law, medicine, education and architecture. These fields offer more flexible forms of upward growth in companies that are less pyramid-shaped than most and a kind of job satisfaction that is less dependent on promotions.

Today more than ever, degrees count in the race to the top. The days of being able to rise like Horatio Alger from the mailroom to the boardroom are gone, a result of the trimming of middle-management positions that functioned as rungs for the upwardly mobile man. "On average, higher education equals higher pay," says Ken Hoyt, Ph.D., a Kansas State University career development specialist. More and more CEOs of the future are going to have degrees behind their names.

Do You Really Want to Claw?

You also might want to ask yourself if the corporate climb is worth the effort for you. Clawing your way to the top is a lifestyle choice that involves much sacrifice. One 42-year-old manager at a steel extrusion plant in Illinois struggled for years to attain a top managerial post, only to find he didn't fit the mold once he got there. He hated dealing with the "people problems" his new post was responsible for. Ultimately, his frustration cost him his marriage, so he transferred to a small computer-software consulting firm where he could get his feet back on the ground. He has felt like a new man ever since. "I can smile again," he says.

Getting off the promotion path may not mean taking a financial beating. If you're good at your job, you'll get paid for it, says Columbia University business professor David Lewin, Ph.D. More and more companies are realizing the importance of keeping key people—even though they won't be able to promote them. Some firms have designed special tracks that offer independence and generous financial rewards—but may never lead to a title change. Given the choice, many men find it easy to sacrifice prestige for the satisfaction of having a life outside their career. "We may find ourselves moving back to a time when work wasn't such an exclusive source of gratification," says Beth King of the Center for Career and Life Planning at New York University.

Society still places great value on reaching the top of the heap, and it's risky to go against the grain. But if anyone can succeed in defying the standard, it's the members of the current generation. As one corporate consultant observes, "The baby boomers place creativity and self-expression at the center of their being."

"People who went through the Great Depression could resign themselves to finishing out their careers on a down note, but baby boomers are more willing to take chances because they expect more from life," says Al Hafer.

But maybe IBM physicist Philip Seiden puts it best. "If you haven't made it in society's eyes, who cares?" asks the 56-year-old, who withdrew from a senior management position 15 years ago to concentrate on research. "Have you made it in *your* eyes? That's what really matters. If you're happy, why strive for more? To satisfy your mother-in-law?"

—Ron Heitzgebot

Corporate Blunders

FYI: Nine ways to assure yourself of failure. Here's an executive's guide to slipping up (and how to avoid it).

Step into any mall bookstore and you'll find a dozen volumes on how to achieve nearly supernatural success at work. Donald Trump, Lee Iacocca, the guy with the weird hair who bought the shaver company—they've all been more than happy to share their secrets on how to make the big coin.

But where are the books for the man who wants to flee from success, who longs to *fail?* Why isn't there a manual of reverse alchemy for guys who desire to turn their gold medals into lead? Apparently there's a big audience waiting out there.

"Fear of success is common," says Mortimer Feinberg, Ph.D., chairman of BFS Psychological Associates, a New York management consulting firm. "It's the desire to get away from the pressures of achievement. Each new success is seen by some men as a new enslavement. One way to bail out of the increased responsibilities is to fail."

Other men, he says, feel unworthy of good fortune. They regard themselves as losers and look for ways to prove it. Hand one of them the reins and he'll strive to wrap them around his neck.

"When people with low self-esteem succeed, they feel like frauds, so they sabotage their success," Dr. Feinberg explains. "Their policy is: It's better to sit in the back of the room and be discovered than to sit at the front of the room and be found out."

If you have a subtle urge to fail because of an aversion to responsibility or anemic self-esteem, Dr. Feinberg has done your homework for you. He interviewed a dozen top executives who were willing to share, anonymously, the secrets of their major screw-ups. *Now these proven failure techniques can be yours!* Consider them ammunition for shooting yourself in the foot. Of course, if failure is *not* what you have in mind, this guide can serve as a rundown of behaviors to resist.

Refuse to share your power. Insist on exclusive control and don't bother to solicit opinions, so that any flops are entirely to your discredit. "You won't survive long as an autocrat," Dr. Feinberg says. He cites the blunder of a young executive in a food-distributing company who was so enamored of a new yogurt-and-nut product that he didn't consult his sales staff before ordering boxcar-loads. Then he discovered his salespeople hated the stuff and would have gladly told him so if he'd asked. "He and his family were eating the yogurt for years," Dr. Feinberg says.

The converse of this is the survival strategy of David Dubinsky, the former head of the International Ladies' Garment Workers Union. "When things go right, I make the decisions," Dubinsky said. "When things go wrong, I look for a partner."

Organize the opposition. When you beat out a colleague for a promotion, make sure he stays an opponent. If you lose, hold a grudge. Never join forces with your rivals.

Lyndon Johnson was savvy enough to avoid this blunder, says Dr. Feinberg. "If he lost to an adversary, he sought reconciliation. That's why after challenging Kennedy for the presidential nomination, he could take second place on the ticket and go on to become president himself. And whenever he won, he was wise enough to bring the defeated rival into camp. He once said of J. Edgar Hoover, a potential adversary, 'I'd rather have him inside the tent pissing out than outside the tent pissing in.'"

Or as former baseball manager Leo Durocher once said, "I never let the four guys who hate me get together with the five who are undecided."

Be arrogant and treat your staff like hired hands. You'll quickly demotivate people, cripple their effectiveness, and turn potential friends into enemies. "Charles Revson of Revlon had a deserved reputation for a dictatorial attitude," says Dr. Feinberg. "He had a large security staff because he was afraid competitors would find a way to steal his product secrets. One time, a new security guard asked him for his pass and he instantly fired her. He said, 'She should have known who I am.' "

Adds Dr. Feinberg: "One of the executives at Estée Lauder claimed he staffed the Lauder company with refugees. 'From Germany?' someone asked. 'No, from Revlon,' he said."

Once you've made it to the top, disregard the people who put you there. Dr. Feinberg interviewed one executive with a strong record of achievements who tended to keep his board of directors waiting rather than interrupt his own tasks. His healthy bottom line didn't save him from getting booted in the end.

"Ignoring those who helped you rather than staying in loyal contact with them builds a lot of animosity," says Dr. Feinberg. "This turned out to be one of the most common errors of those who failed."

Defer all painful judgments regarding personnel. Wait until a disaster strikes to make the inevitable decision to fire that nice, incompetent person on your staff.

Take big financial risks for relatively small rewards. "When you get carried away by your own grandiosity, you forget the risk-to-reward ratio," says Dr. Feinberg. He gives the example of a manager who devotes a lot of his company's resources to cutting into a small, competitive market with a new product. "Even if the product succeeds, his company isn't going to make much, and if it flops, there's going to be a big loss."

Cling to a product or service beyond its heyday. Insist that your product, your baby, is immune to the market's life cycles. Dr. Feinberg points to the American automobile industry in the 1970s producing outmoded gas guzzlers while a squadron of Japanese compacts whizzed by in the fast lane.

Release a product or service before it's ready. If your idea is so hot it's practically radioactive, why let those drones in market research and production hold things up with their boring calculations?

Go for broke—literally. One computer company announced an improved model prematurely, says Dr. Feinberg. Customers passed up the current version and waited for the better one. But the new model hit production snags and wasn't ready on time. Cash flow dribbled to a stop, and the company went belly-up.

Ignore your competitors. If your business is on a roll, don't keep looking over your shoulder at the other guys. You'll coast downhill. "The Swiss were shown some of the early digital watch designs, but they didn't want to make them. They said, 'It's not a watch—it doesn't have springs and gears.' They didn't think digital watches would put a dent in their market," says Dr. Feinberg.

By practicing even a few of these failure techniques, almost any executive can soon turn his throne of command into an ejection seat. Carefully avoid these pitfalls, and one day someone might ask you to write a book about how to get to the top.

—Peter Keely

The Essence of Control

Ever wonder how you might get control over your job, your stress, your time . . . your life? Here are the answers.

You spend more time at work than you do asleep in your own bed. Where once you whispered sweet nothings in your wife's ear, you now exchange urgent information: "Did you pay the electric bill?" "Did the recyclable trash go out?" "Did the plumber get the Little Mermaid doll out of the drain?" Your daughter has taken to fantasizing that she is Shirley Temple, and you're her long-lost father, missing in action in the Boer War.

This is not the life you set out to lead. It is, instead, a life careening wildly out of control, a life with a life of its own.

If this sounds familiar, it may not be your fault. Most of us are working more hours, and for all our toil in the corporate vineyard, our efforts don't always bear fruit. Our earnings are in a race with our expenses, and the expenses are winning. And because we have to work more just to keep even, free time is at a premium. Welcome to the 1990s.

"The average workweek has just exploded, to an average of over 46 hours," says time-management consultant and author Merrill Douglass. "I know managers and professionals who are working 50 and 60 hours. Top-level people often put in 60 to 70 hours, on average. We have millions of people out there whose lives consist of eating, sleeping, household maintenance and working, and I think they're hurting."

Welcome to Chaos

Of course, you don't need a sour economy or a family to feel powerless in the face of daily responsibilities. Even in the best of times, your life may be chaotic. But the recent recession and the continuing financial difficulties underscore what is likely to be an important continuing theme in American life: the loss of control, and the need for more of it.

However, you *can* get your life back in order. Not just your work life, but your whole life. You can get control of your time so you have more of it to spend with family, friends and by yourself. You can get control of the mounting stress so you have more peace of mind. And you can get control of your diet and exercise plans as well. Better still, you can achieve this kind of control by making a series of small changes.

The essence of control is a feeling, say the experts. You can't influence the outcome of every event in your life, explains clinical psychologist Ronald Nathan, Ph.D., coauthor of *The Doctors' Guide To Instant Stress Relief.* But you can *feel* in control. He describes this quality as an emotional hardiness, an almost chameleon-like adaptability.

This hardiness, he believes, is rooted in a sense of purpose. Purpose means having overriding goals, a comprehensive plan for your life that will see you through good times and bad. People who have this kind of long-range vision are able to see temporary setbacks for what they are; they know where they're going, and they aren't going to let anything stand in the way. "It all stems from a belief that you have real influence over what happens in your life through what you imagine, say or do," says Suzanne Ouellette Kobasa, Ph.D., a professor of psychology at the graduate school of the City University of New York.

A Sense of Purpose Is Key

You can't instantaneously attain that belief. But even if it seems like your daily routine is an exercise in damage control, somewhere deep down you need a sense of purpose, or the tools necessary to find it. Douglass, owner of Time Management Center in Marietta, Georgia, and coauthor of *Manage Your Time, Manage Your Work, Manage Yourself,* recommends following a clear and well-defined action plan that'll help you regain your sense of purpose and give you back your control.

To begin with, keep a journal in which you jot down what you do in every hour, in your work, family and personal life for a month. Once you've developed this sample one-month life map, look at the things that you spend your time doing and separate them into things you love doing and things you don't. Then ask yourself: How much time do I spend doing the things I really want to do with my life? How can I rearrange my life to get more of what I want?

The experts stress that in identifying your desires, what you should be looking for are the kinds of things that would make you feel happy and fulfilled. This does not include short-term, transitory goals, like "Make megabucks" or "Become vice-president of the company," but rather things like "I want to work in a helping profession" or "I want to have more time in my life to be with my family."

"Once you've found that answer, the rest is relatively easy," says Douglass. "We spend so much time running around trying to figure out what to do. But we need to figure out what we want to *be* first."

Hardy people, those whom Dr. Nathan describes as in control of their lives, committed to goals and challenged by change, have one other telling characteristic: flexibility. They roll with the punches. They don't waste time trying to change what they can't change. "They have the ability to recognize when it's time to pull back or when they don't have control," says Dr. Ouellette Kobasa. "They're better able to tolerate ambiguity. People who don't feel in control just can't tolerate it when the world becomes unpredictable, as it often is."

Forget Fear of Failure

"A lot of our stress has to do with failed expectations," adds Dr. Nathan, pointing out what may seem an obvious fact, but one we must all take to heart: "The world isn't set up to meet our expectations. We'd all be better off if we could remember that."

One of the major approaches to reducing stress, he adds, is to examine what your expectations are. If you expect to fix the garage-door opener, play golf, get a haircut and pick up your laundry all in one Saturday afternoon, you're going to feel out of control. Likewise, business and professional goals also need to be challenging but not out of reach. "And we have to change our expectations as the world changes," he says. "Often, our expectations lag behind where the world really is."

Sometimes circumstances really are overwhelming. There's too much to do, and not enough time to do it all. So you either adapt, or you find ways to reduce the pressures that are making you feel less than fully in control. Some general principles apply.

Take Little Bites

First, don't bite off more than you can chew. Sounds simple, but it isn't always. Some men just can't say no. They have their fingers in every little pie, from negotiating multimillion-dollar contracts to choosing the color of the new office telephones. They do charity work. They're on the company softball team. They don't know how to stop.

Robert Dato, Ph.D., is a Wynnewood, Pennsylvania, psychoanalyst who helps executives learn to adapt to stress. He says he often sees men who are in way over their heads. "They come in and they tell me all the things they're doing. I try to understand all the pressures they don't need to be under," Dr. Dato says. He helps them decide what's best for them, which usually means reducing pressure and increasing adaptability in stressful situations. "When they do this, they get great relief, but it's like they need the permission of a therapist, a father figure," says Dr. Dato. "I tell them it's okay."

Of course, you don't need a therapist to tell you when you're doing too much. You probably already know. Nor should you need anyone's permission but your own. If you can't go cold turkey, try dropping one activity at a time until the pressure's off.

It may be easy to drop all your extracurricular activities, but it's not so simple to tell your boss you just don't feel like doing accounts payable today. Still, even at work, there are ways to extricate yourself tactfully when you're overloaded. If you do it with enough skill, says Dr. Nathan, your boss will think you're saying no for his own good: "Say, 'I'm overcommitted, and I can't really do that justice,' " Dr. Nathan recommends. "Say, 'I'm flattered that you asked, but I wouldn't want to agree to do something for you if I really didn't have the time to do a good job.' "

Another approach, for bosses with harder heads, is to offer options, says Douglass. "Tell him, 'I'd really like to do this for you, but

NEAT LITTLE TIMESAVERS

Here are some nifty tricks to help you gain better control of your life.

• Hang a key rack near the front door and make it a habit to put your keys there as soon as you walk in. You'll never again have to frantically search for them when you're already running late.

• Get up 15 minutes earlier in the morning. Then, if anything goes wrong, you won't have to deal with being late on top of it. Likewise, plan to leave 15 minutes earlier than you usually do for appointments so you won't have to rush.

• Lay out your clothes, fill the coffee machine and check your briefcase before you go to bed. Mornings are so much easier when all the details are arranged.

• Pay all your bills on the same day each month. Ideally this should be the same day you get your bank statement, so you can reconcile it at the same time. File all bills that arrive after this date in a central location to be paid next month.

• Use pickup and delivery services whenever possible. You'll save time, and in many cases you'll save money as well when you take into account the cost of driving to get the paper or the dry cleaning.

I can't do it without giving up something else. Which of these things would you most like me to do?' Most bosses will take the hint."

Get Fit

Along with emotional hardiness, physical fitness can go a long way toward improving your sense of well-being. Clearly, exercise benefits the body and makes you hardier, says Dr. Ouellette Kobasa, but she adds, "It has something to do, too, with what's going on in your head. People who can get up from their desks and take a ten-minute walk feel better about themselves than those people who say, 'I can't ever leave my desk.' That ten minutes of walking is just for you. It is also a time for some reflection. While you're out walking, you can see a problem for

• Set priorities. Write your day's tasks, in order of importance, on a series of sticky notes. When you complete a task, peel off the note and crumple it up with a feeling of accomplishment.

• Avoid business lunches when possible. Use the time as a psychological break, a time to balance out the morning and afternoon.

• Use a tape recorder for your correspondence. It's twice as efficient as dictation or longhand.

• To make Mondays easier, take the last hour of every Friday to straighten up your office. Write reminders to yourself for Monday morning. Also, save a couple of your more pleasurable tasks for Monday.

• The average executive wastes 288 hours a year in unnecessary meetings. Go into meetings with a clear objective. Beforehand, ask yourself questions like "Do I need to reach a decision about something?" "Do I want to share information?" Ask yourself if you could handle things in a memo or by phone more easily.

• Plan a way to avoid interruptions. Set aside a time each day when you can work without distraction. Make sure everyone on your staff knows when that time is. Then close the door.

what it is, and you often come back with a much better perspective."

Exercise done outside of work is also very helpful, she says, because it puts you into contact with other people. Social support is another key element in the development of that elusive thing called hardiness. "The human organism is a complex thing," she says, "and we're more resistant to stress when we have this combination of social, psychological and biological factors working in our favor."

One unscheduled activity that intrudes on your sense of well-being throughout the day is worry. And the more you worry, the more you feel that you're not in control. Worry overwhelms all reason. And even as you budget time for work and play, worry has free rein. One solution, recommends Dr. Nathan, is to set aside a formal time each day for worry.

"Sometimes we worry superstitiously, as if worrying will control the future," Dr. Nathan says. "People are under the illusion that they're somehow planning what to do. But are they planning or worrying?"

If you're really planning, he suggests that you pull out the pad and pencil and write down what you're going to do. But if you're really just worrying, nothing's being accomplished. You're giving yourself a false sense of control.

Schedule Your Worrying

Research suggests that setting aside time for worry—a half hour toward the end of each day—actually decreases the amount of worry by an average of 35 percent, thus increasing your sense of well-being.

Finally, whenever you're able, try to accentuate the positive. So maybe your Alfa-Romeo needs a $1,100 transmission job. Maybe the kids need braces and your cat is allergic to fleas. Okay, so the IRS has sent you a notice that you're being audited. All true, and all pretty gruesome. On the other hand, you're healthy. Your marriage is good. Your kids think you're God and you could *afford* the fancy car in the first place. "The key," says Dr. Nathan, "is to identify areas of your life where you *do* have control."

In the meantime, hang in there. As someone once said, you can't smooth out the surf, but you can learn to ride the waves.

—*Jeff Meade*

Execu-Pains

As if you didn't know, the repressed urge to punch or kick somebody results in muscular stresses. If that somebody happens to be at your place of work, here's what to do.

Dave Howard is one of the most stressed-out people I know, and I know a *lot* of stressed-out people. In the past five years, Dave has had three middle-management jobs shot out from under him for reasons beyond his control. And each job seems more stressful than the last. Most recently, he was with the U.S. branch of a Japanese firm. To meet incredibly tight and unforgiving production deadlines, it was essential that he communicate closely with a man who didn't speak very good English. After months of trying to boost the guy's language skills by chatting about women and whatnot, there came a crisis. "I told him the schedule wasn't working, we had to ship in three days, and he was getting way behind," Dave recalls. "I said 'Do you understand?' And he said, 'Girlfriend?'"

Griping about this stuff over a not-so-happy-hour beer helps Dave get through. But it does nothing for the aches he gets all over—in his jaw, neck and shoulders (which often lead to headaches) and in his lower back and legs. Sometimes the pains hit him singly; sometimes they gang up on him. He's a walking—rather, *sitting*—textbook on what Richard M. Bachrach, D.O., calls execu-pains.

As medical director of the Center for Sports and Osteopathic Medicine in New York, Dr. Bachrach sees the same gallery of minor aches and pains all the time among his white-collar clientele. Often the underlying problem is a lack of exercise or bottled-up aggression, he says. "Guys who don't get enough physical activity can't diffuse the energy that builds up from day-to-day frustrations. The repressed urge to punch or kick somebody results directly in muscular stresses, particularly among lower-level executives who have a lot of responsibility, but no control over their jobs."

Clench Your Fist

To get an idea of where neck pain actually comes from, clench your fist and visualize what's going on inside. Muscles are hard, contracted, pressing against the skin. These muscles also push against nerves, and over time those nerves can become irritated, explains Richard M. Linchitz, M.D., medical director of the Pain Alleviation Center in Roslyn, New York. Different people express their tension in different parts of the body. "Some get ulcers, some develop high blood pressure, some will get a heart attack in 20 years—and some get neck pains and tension headaches," says Dr. Linchitz. "In certain people there seems to be a kind of constitutional predisposition—a weakness—to muscular pain."

Often, the weakness stems from an injury (which itself could be stress related—tense muscles are less supple). My friend Dave's problems began when a nerve became pinched by a swollen disk while running. It healed, but slowly. He stopped exercising, which set off a spiraling degeneration: Lack of activity made him more susceptible to stress, which made his back feel worse, which kept him awake nights, which left him exhausted—making his back feel worse. Then the aches and pains began to spread. In severe cases, this kind of progression can lead to a chronic condition called fibromyalgia that lasts for months or years and virtually incapacitates people.

But it needn't be so. "These pains are very interrelated, and we can manage them ourselves, without expensive or time-consuming treatments," says Dr. Bachrach. The best remedy is to relieve the stress itself, either by avoiding anxiety-provoking situations or by tapping a variety of relaxation techniques. But there are also physical ways to soothe pains where they live—in the muscles.

Prescription number one is exercise. "In some cases, working the muscle that's in pain ultimately can be the best thing for it, despite the usual wisdom of not doing something that hurts," Dr. Linchitz says. (But don't push pained muscles too far. It's important that exercises be moderate and properly performed.) Stretching to relieve stiffness can help keep pains from ever hitting, but if you hurt in a particular area, you should perform a therapeutic stretch at least three times a day. Here's a guide to the six most common execu-pains and the simplest, most effective tips for easing them.

Head and Neck Aches

They almost always go together. Common causes are cradling a phone with your shoulder or craning your neck to view a computer screen. That pain in the neck often radiates upward, creating a band of tightness from the base of the skull or around the forehead.

1. Sitting erect in a chair, let your chin fall gently to your chest, allowing the weight of your head to stretch muscles at the back of the neck. Keep the neck relaxed, and hold for 30 seconds. Next, lean your head back gently and look at the ceiling for 30 seconds. (Caution: Older men, 65 years and up, may feel faint or pass out when they do this stretch. Check with your doctor first.)

2. Grip the bottom of the chair you're sitting on with your left hand, so that your left shoulder pulls down slightly, then lean your head gently to the right. Hold for 30 seconds. Repeat, opposite side.

Jaw Soreness

This problem is typically characterized by pain on one side of the face shooting into the head. People under pressure have a tendency to clench and grind their teeth, which can lead to a jaw malady called temporomandibular joint (TMJ) disorder. "But a lot of so-called TMJ problems are really due to muscular tension on one side of the jaw," says Dr. Linchitz. "That creates an imbalance, and the muscle acts as if there's a problem in the joint itself."

1. Open your mouth about halfway and gently swivel the lower jaw right and left, moving it continuously for about 30 seconds.

2. Bring your lower jaw forward and up in front of the upper jaw ten times before a meal and another ten times before bed.

3. To keep from clenching your teeth, hold your jaw open slightly so upper and lower teeth are separated. Rest your tongue lightly against the roof of your mouth without pressing it against the front teeth. With practice, this may become habitual, reducing the urge to clench or grind.

Shoulder Pain

Most shoulder soreness comes from irregular use of or physical abuse to muscles and tendons, but with stress, neck pains can irritate the nerves that lead to the arms, allowing pain to radiate to the shoulders.

1. Bring your left arm in front of your body, across your chest. Hook your right arm under your left elbow and pull your left arm across your chest. Hold for 30 seconds and release. Repeat, opposite side.

2. Raise your left arm straight up and grab the top or side of a door frame. Holding the frame, walk through the door until you feel muscles stretch gently. Hold for 30 seconds and release. Repeat with your right arm.

3. Reach up to your side at a 45-degree angle, taking hold of a door frame with your left hand. Gently twist your body to the right, away from the raised arm. Hold for 30 seconds and release. Repeat with your right arm.

4. Hold one arm straight out to the side, elbow bent at 90 degrees, as if taking an oath. Grab the side of a door frame with your raised hand and walk through the door until muscles stretch gently. Hold for 30 seconds. Release, then repeat with the other arm.

Backaches

The back is particularly vulnerable, because muscles here do most of the work of supporting the body when you're sitting. "If you don't have a good chair, you're dead," says Dave, my stressed-out friend. But even if your company springs for the latest ergonomic wonder, you should change position a lot, stand when you're on the phone and stretch frequently. When pain hits, if it's mild, try these stretches. (For severe back pain, consult your doctor.)

1. Grab the doorknobs on both sides of an open door. Keeping your arms straight in front of you and your feet flat on the floor, squat as low as you can while pulling on the knobs. Hold for 30 seconds, then stand up. Caution: Don't do this exercise if you have bad knees.

2. While sitting in your chair, grab one knee with both hands and bring it to your chest. Hold for 15 to 30 seconds. Repeat with the other knee.

Leg Pain

Pain often starts in the lower back and shoots downward. Leg pains are often called sciatica, a condition that may signal serious problems from a herniated disk. However, more than 90 percent of sciatica-like pain isn't true sciatica, but minor pain (usually in the buttocks and upper leg) caused by prolonged sitting. (Don't get alarmed unless the pain extends below the knee or persists for several days.)

To stretch buttocks muscles, sit erect in a chair and cross your left leg over your right, ankle-on-knee. Cup your left knee with your left hand and your left ankle with your right hand. Simultaneously pull your knee and ankle toward your right shoulder until you feel muscles stretch slightly. Hold for 30 seconds and release. Repeat with your right leg.

Stretches like these helped get Dave back on track. For his particular problem, his doctor also recommended taking up swimming, an activity that doesn't strain his still-sensitive back. He'll always be nervous about job security, but he's now comfortably ensconced in a stable wing of a stable company. He says his pains are becoming less frequent and less intense. The stress is still there, but he had to hang up before he could finish telling me about it: His boss was coming and he didn't want to have to explain exactly what he was doing talking to a reporter on company time.

—*Richard Laliberte*

John Henry Had It Wrong

If you believe that simply putting your nose to the grindstone will allow you to succeed, take a lesson from the man who died trying.

By now, most of us have found out that there's no such thing as an A for effort. In the real world of real work, effort doesn't count a whole lot in the absence of results. Still, the notion that we'll always be rewarded for working hard is one that some men carry with them all their lives. It's all mixed up with popular American myths about rising from rags to riches, from some humble shanty to the White House. "I can do anything," we're encouraged to believe. "The sky's the limit."

Social scientists have come up with a name for this kind of hard-work-beats-all reasoning: *John Henryism.*

You remember the story: John Henry was the best steel-driving man on the railroad. When a machine came along to do his job, he swore he could outperform steam power any day. In a contest, John Henry indeed beat the machine, but then collapsed with a ruptured blood vessel in his head. Not exactly a clear victory.

Today, John Henry is the middle manager who sets out irrationally to leapfrog a grade level in the company by adding projects to a plate that's already too full. He's the entrepreneur who resolves this

285

year to crack a business market that's long resisted his best efforts. He's the man who sets out to buy a house he can barely afford, despite a downturn in his business.

"John Henry epitomizes a spirit of hard work and determination against all odds," says E. C. McKetney, Ph.D., an epidemiologist at the University of California, Berkeley. "And John Henryism is a belief that simply putting your nose to the grindstone and doing things on your own will allow you to succeed no matter what."

Never Saying No

It's not just working hard that makes for a John Henry. It can also be striving unrealistically for goals that you lack the money, the time, the talent or even the social connections to accomplish.

Over time, this approach to the world can kill you just as it did the man the syndrome was named after. The stress of working long hours and never saying no in situations where you can't make a difference may eventually wreck your mental or physical health, says Salvatore Maddi, Ph.D., professor of psychology at the University of California, Irvine, and president of the Hardiness Institute, a stress-management firm.

Studies find that stress plays a role in the onset of 90 percent of mental disorders, and some medical professionals estimate that 60 percent of all visits to a doctor are stress related. "You use up your body's resources, and your immune system turns to mush," Dr. Maddi says. Wearing down the body eventually can hasten the progress of life-threatening problems such as heart disease and cancer. Studies among low-income, uneducated, rural blacks—people whose resources for accomplishing their goals are especially low—find that men who believe most strongly that hard work and determination will overcome obstacles have higher rates of hypertension than men who are more laid back.

How can you tell if you're a John Henry? According to Sherman James, Ph.D., the University of Michigan epidemiologist who created the John Henryism concept, you'll have a bedrock of certain core attitudes. When the going gets tough, a John Henry wants to work harder, and will stick with a job until it's completely done, always managing to find a way to do the things he really needs to get done. In the face of setbacks, he *never* loses sight of his goals. He's fiercely individualistic, likes doing things that other people thought couldn't be done—and doing them his way. He may also be a little bit overbearing, sometimes feeling that he's the only one who can do a job right.

Overcoming Insecurity

Ironically, these very qualities, in moderation, are what lead to career success. "Managers love people like that," observes Howard Mase, Ph.D., a vice-president at Metropolitan Life Personal Insurance. "They stay all hours, work on weekends, do things nobody else will and don't like to take vacations." Like John Henry himself, they're willing to keep pounding away at problems, even if it kills them.

There's nothing inherently troublesome about having a hard-work ethic, Dr. James says. Problems start when it's combined with unreasonable ambition.

"If these men accomplish one set of goals, they set higher ones," says Stephen Weinstein, Ph.D., clinical professor of psychiatry and human behavior at Thomas Jefferson University Medical College in Philadelphia. "It's an endless cycle, and they never feel they accomplish much of anything. The result is stress, disappointment and frustration."

Psychologists say men often work hard just for the sake of work because they don't feel good about themselves if they're not productive. Deep down, it may have to do with feelings they got from their parents that their worth in the world is measured by what they do, not by who they are. Working hard, according to this view, becomes a way for them to control affection and gain the admiration of other people.

In this respect, John Henry types bear a resemblance to people with Type-A personalities, whose hard-driving, aggressive and often hostile behavior make them particularly stress-prone. John Henrys lack many of the hallmark Type-A characteristics—they're not likely to express anger forcefully, for example—but both personalities have an overwhelming need for absolute control over their lives, says Dr. Maddi. "For them to assess a situation and say 'I can't do anything' is the worst thing in the world for them," he says. "They'll never reach that conclusion. They'll just try harder. The trouble is they won't always be successful."

Finding Peace

Consider the case of Lee Atwater, the late chairman of the Republican Party. When he learned he had inoperable cancer, the 39-

year-old Atwater marshalled his staff and instructed them to explore every possibility for finding a cure. He was determined that the disease would not beat him. Whether his frustration hastened his death is anybody's guess, but eventually he came to terms with the fact that the matter was out of his hands. That, according to his own account, is when he began to find some peace.

So it is with the rest of us, psychologists say. What we need—and what John Henrys lack—is to accept that yes, we can accomplish a lot by dint of our own effort, but some obstacles in life are as immovable as the Rockies. So instead of butting your head against the stone, go around it. Instead of working so hard to overcome your weaknesses, start doing more things that accentuate your strengths.

How do you know when a goal is unrealistic? It sounds trite, but you won't know until you try. "Goals should always be challenging," says Cliff Mangan, Ph.D., a psychologist at Temple University Counseling Center in Philadelphia. "But you have to ask yourself if what you're doing is getting you toward that goal."

If your goal is to rise two grade levels in your company, break your approach into smaller, more manageable goals—rising first to the next-highest level, for example, or cultivating the social contacts that may boost your ascent. Give yourself a specific, reasonable amount of time for these developments to occur.

If your efforts don't seem to pay off, try another approach, such as getting more training or education, suggests Dr. Maddi. "Persistence can be helpful, but you need to see clearly what can be changed and what can't," he says. When you run out of ideas, it's time to get out of the steam engine's way and find something else to challenge.

—Richard Laliberte

Surviving Success

A counselor to the rich and powerful tells how to keep from hitting bottom when you reach the top.

You expect to make a few sacrifices on your way to the top. The hope is that you'll be more than compensated for the price of success when you reach that big payoff at the peak.

However, many men discover that the cost is just too steep. They've reaped material rewards, but feel they've been emotionally swindled in the process. "Success is one of the most psychologically disruptive experiences a person can endure," says Steven Berglas, Ph.D., a clinical psychologist and management consultant at Harvard Medical School, and author of *The Success Syndrome: Hitting Bottom When You Reach the Top.*

It's largely a matter of feeling isolated from other people, says Dr. Berglas, and the more successful you are, the less likely it is that others will take your emotional needs seriously.

Is it possible to reach your career goals with your emotional health intact? Dr. Berglas says yes. In his practice at the Executive Stress Clinic in Chestnut Hill, Massachusetts, he counsels achievers on their problems and how to overcome them. We asked him to share some of his insights.

Q. It seems as though people don't have a good understanding of what success is really like. What are some myths about success?

A. The major myth is that career success will transform your personal life. People honestly believe that if they are good at their job they will have friends and lovers as a result. There is no correlation. In fact, there's an antagonism between achieving career success and achieving emotional satisfaction. The skills and attributes necessary for one contradict the other.

Q. Why is that?

A. The traditional route to the top is through the acquisition of wealth and power, not affection. When clients start therapy, I try to get them to discover how they came to depend on financial rewards to secure all forms of gratification. Then we explore what I call the Law of Inverse Business Effects: how actions that advance careers—using the backs of others as stepping stones, for example, or choosing friends on the basis of what they'll do for your career—typically derail relationships.

Highly successful people are often prone to severe bouts of depression. They have an overwhelming sense of emptiness and isolation. If you feel all you've got going for you is money, then everyone around you, including your spouse, seems to be after you for what you can give them rather than who you are. Having no real interpersonal relationships has incredibly devastating effects psychologically.

Q. What are some other problems that go along with success?

A. There's a "halo effect," where the person who's successful in one realm is presumed competent and talented in all others. That generates inordinate expectations, and people really aren't equipped to live up to them. Buzz Aldrin is one of my favorite examples. He had a nervous breakdown after walking on the moon. He was a great astronaut and a great military man, but a horrible hero. He was uncomfortable around people. He was overwhelmed by the social adoration, the expectation that he also could be an after-dinner speaker or chairman of the board.

Another belief about success is that if you do "X" today, you should be able to do "X plus one" tomorrow. It's a constant upward spiral of expectations that no human can live up to. But for men who are dependent on success for their identity, there's no quitting. Ultimately, they'll sacrifice relationships to focus more energy on their careers.

Q. How do people come to recognize these problems in themselves?

A. Let's speak in terms of physical warning signs. The first thing people do is self-medicate—they'll drink more coffee and alcohol, take sleeping aids and often try harder drugs, trying to provide themselves with an "up." The second symptom is an irritability with the family. The third is adultery, as individuals blame partners for their failure to feel upbeat about life. The fourth symptom is trying to seek adventure—buying a Jet Ski or doing an adventurous trip like Outward Bound, for example. When those magic bullets don't work, often they come to psychotherapy and realize there's been a dearth of appropriate rewards.

Q. You've written that this often takes place between the age of 38 and 42. What's so special about that time in a man's life?

A. When I say that, I'm talking about fast-trackers. People in the middle lane would experience this around 50. It's whenever material reinforcers lose their value. You find it does no good to buy a new Rolex or a new Mercedes or a new boat. You just run out of toys. And at the same time you're losing your taste for material things, you discover your inability to achieve emotional and personal satisfaction. It's when you realize you've gotten there and it ain't what it's cracked up be.

Promotions are often a trigger. People assume a promotion will change everything—that now they'll have time for their wife, they'll be a better father, they'll go back to playing basketball at the YMCA and they'll finally feel great.

Nothing of the sort happens. Their interpersonal relationships don't improve, and their anxieties get worse because they have to live up to more expectations. The money and perks make no difference. They move into the corner office, wake up two weeks later and find nothing has improved.

Q. So are you saying there are no benefits to being a success?

A. Not at all. Successful men have opportunities that others do not. If you can clear up your debts, feel secure that your job won't be taken away and aren't concerned with basic self-preservation in your career, you can begin to look at who you are and where you fit into the world. This kind of security allows you to explore relationships, develop your spirituality, figure out where you stand in the world and what it's all about. It's wonderful to be successful if you take advantage of the opportunities you've created.

Q. What does it take to reach the top and stay psychologically healthy?

A. In the studies I've done, the people who are healthy when they reach the top have a strong cultural or religious involvement. I didn't expect to find this church component, but it really is there. They don't necessarily believe strongly in God or the tenets of a church. They don't say the rosary or don't keep a kosher home, but they believe in Catholicism, believe in Judaism, believe in their ethnic heritage.

They also have an intact family and they engage in some form of mentoring. There's a sense of wanting to bring others along, a sense of nurturing, of being a giver. They engage in volunteerism that takes hands-on "sweat equity" in a project, not just saying, "Here's $100,000, put my name on a building." They're very involved, but they don't need monuments.

Q. Can you cite some examples of men who have actually done this?

A. The best one is Peter Lynch of the Magellan Fund. Richest guy on Wall Street and walks away to spend time with his wife and daughters. He's also involved with the church and the alumni association at Boston College. Another example is Thomas Monaghan of Domino's Pizza. He's one of the richest men in America, and he's cutting back in his midforties to do missionary work for the church.

Q. What else can we do on the way up?

A. The major thing I advocate is systematically trading off material gratifications for interpersonal rewards. If a move will take you away from a place where you're starting to root and to develop a social net-work, pass up the 10 percent raise and realize you're being paid back in other ways. If a promotion involves travel and you don't want to travel, pass up the promotion. Another one will come along.

I also advocate entering organizations outside your work where you can be an "Indian," not a "chief." It's no good being an executive in a community softball league if you're also an executive at work—it isn't going to permit you to develop the interpersonal contacts that make you feel good about who you are. But when you're a drone, people come to know you as a person. Peer groups like the Young Presidents Organization can have the same effect because members can relate to one another as people—everybody's as rich as everybody else, so they're not there for the hustle.

Q. What about family life? Do the same principles apply?

A. Exactly. I see plenty of high-powered types who don't know how to stop behaving like executives. They come home, sit at the dining room table and hold a board meeting, with progress reports from each child as though he were a little subsidiary. This is probably the biggest problem they confront. They have to learn to be a peer in the family, not always a superstar, to abandon competency as a method of gain-ing intimacy.

The easiest way to do it is through what's called a "strategic pratfall effect." You need to show vulnerability to your kids and your spouse.

Tell a child, "I'm afraid of those computers you're learning with" or "I don't know that foreign language you're studying." When your son comes to you to talk about his fears, don't say, "You need to be strong like me." That's another distancing technique. It intimidates him and tells him that it's not okay to be human. Instead say, "When I was your age, this was something I went through."

You have to differentiate *liking*, which you want from your family, from *respect*, which you want from your colleagues. You don't tell your colleagues you're scared. You definitely tell your kids.

Q. What's the moral of the story?

A. Love and work are the key to mental health, and in America we've really denigrated the role of love. By love I mean love of God, love of community, love of principles, love of people. Romantic love, too.

I advise tons of companies to let their young executives teach, mentor, get involved with community outreach. The corporation will be polishing its image better than any media consultant would, and the executives will feel more like people. This would be a tremendous benefit.

—*Richard Laliberte*

PART 11

Ask *Men's Health*

30 Questions Men Ask Most

From nutrition to sex to hair loss to beer— here are the answers to the questions nearly every guy has asked at least once in his life. In case you haven't—it's about time you did!

Pouring Beer

Q. I've noticed that bartenders always pour beer down the side of the glass to keep the foam down. But I've heard that it's better to pour the beer into the center of the glass because this helps to unlock the flavor. Is there any merit to this theory?

—C.J., Tallahassee, Florida

A. There is. By pouring beer into the center of the glass, you get more bubbles, which release the aroma of the beer and enhance its taste, according to Charlie Papazian, president of the American Homebrewers Association. On the other hand, you don't want to put too much of a head on your beer. Optimum pouring is a matter of balance, says Papazian. He suggests you begin by letting the beer flow down the side of the glass, then move the stream into the center in order to top off the beer with a half-inch head.

Bashful Bladder

Q. Since college, I've had a problem urinating in nervous situations and crowded public places. Even when I'm totally relaxed, my urine flow starts weak before getting stronger. It's become a terrible burden, and I need to know if something can be done. Can you recommend any medical procedures? Could this be totally mental?

—*J.L., Philadelphia, Pennsylvania*

A. You've got what doctors call bashful bladder syndrome—a condition that we've all experienced at one time or another. What happens is that something makes you uneasy, and as a result, you involuntarily tense up the muscles that control the flow of urine out of your bladder. A lot of things can set this problem off—even just having the boss walk up to the next urinal. What complicates it all is worrying that it'll happen again. Then you get in a vicious cycle: Because you're worried, you tense up and can't pee. Because you can't pee, you're still worried, and so on.

It's not, in any case, a serious problem, since the pressure of the urine in your bladder will eventually overwhelm the muscles trying to hold it back. When the problem is at its worst, the easiest solution is to just wait for a stall in the bathroom. Funny how a little privacy makes all the difference.

You can overcome bashful bladder syndrome by learning how to consciously relax those muscles, say the experts. Practice stopping and starting your urine flow—in the privacy of your own bathroom, of course. If the problem is really a burden as you say, a psychiatrist can prescribe drugs to help relax those troublesome muscles.

The Extra Stretch

Q. I've read that stretching after running can help keep my muscles more flexible. I stretch for at least ten minutes after every run, but my body never seems to get any more elastic. Am I doing something wrong, or was I just born stiff?

—*B.A., Mountain View, California*

A. Stretching after a run is only enough to counteract the muscle tightening that occurred during that run, says Pat Croce, physical conditioning coach for Philadelphia's 76ers and Flyers. If you want to really loosen up, you need to throw in some extra stretches at various times during the day. One of the easiest ways to work stretching into your schedule is to do a few minutes after you get up in the morning and a few more before going to bed. To avoid pulling a cold muscle, never bounce and always do at least two sets of each stretch—working up to 60 seconds per stretch.

Where Do I Apply Cologne?

Q. What's the right amount of cologne to use, and where should I apply it?

—*A.M., Phoenix, Arizona*

A. The most common mistake men make with cologne is that they splash it on their faces, says Annette Green, director of the Fragrance Foundation in New York City. That not only dries out facial skin, because of the alcohol that's mixed in with the fragrance, but also tends to result in too much of a good thing. You probably already know which of your coworkers are splashing on cologne; you can smell them coming around the corner.

Proper cologne use requires more subtlety. Put a few drops on your fingertips, then dab lightly behind each ear with your fingers. If you want to live dangerously, rub a little on the center of your chest as well. Wash your hands with soap and warm water before going out—fragrant handshakes won't win you any points with business associates.

For the office, Green recommends lighter types of cologne, which are dominated by smells of citrus, mint or spice. Save heavier fragrances like musk, floral or woodsy scents for after hours. If you're not sure which is which, ask a salesperson at the fragrance counter.

Finally, even following these guidelines, you're going to run into problems if you use cologne with a different brand of scented shaving cream or after-shave. You'll end up with what fragrance-business people call "clashing scents."

Ready-to-Use Eyeglasses Okay?

Q. Lately, I've been having difficulty reading the fine type in some newspapers, so I've started wearing a pair of ready-to-use reading glasses I found at a pharmacy. Any danger in this?

—*A.H., Palacios, Texas*

A. Not as far as we can see. According to our experts, ready-to-use reading glasses are a safe and inexpensive way to correct a common kind of farsightedness known as presbyopia. It's caused when the lenses in our eyes begin to lose some of their elasticity, making it harder to focus on close-up objects. The problem usually becomes noticeable sometime around your fortieth birthday. Typically, you find yourself holding reading matter farther and farther away from your eyes. It's time for glasses when your arms aren't long enough to bring the type into focus.

To select the right pair of reading glasses, hold a newspaper at normal reading distance as you try on several pairs in ascending order of strength. There are 16 different levels of magnification, ranging from +1.00 (the weakest) to +4.00 (the strongest), and the glasses should be identified by these numbers on their hang tags. You'll know you've found the right pair when the print becomes clear and stays that way while you read for several minutes.

Should you begin to experience headaches or tired eyes while reading with your glasses, it's possible you have an underlying vision disorder that requires prescription lenses or treatment from an ophthalmologist. Ask your family doctor for a referral.

Low Ejaculate Volume

Q. I'm 38 years old, and over the past year I've noticed that my second and third ejaculations, even over several hours, produce very little semen. Although I had a vasectomy six years ago, I hadn't noticed any difference until now. Could that have anything to do with my problem? How can I restore the volume of my youth?

—*C.O., Pasadena, California*

A. Your vasectomy has nothing to do with it. The operation only blocks the release of sperm, which account for a very small percentage of the volume of the ejaculate.

As you get older, your body simply doesn't produce as much semen as it used to. So seeing some decline in the volume of your ejaculate is no surprise, especially if you're talking about multiple orgasms, says E. Douglas Whitehead, M.D., a director of the Association for Male Sexual Dysfunction.

There are no magic pills or foods that will increase your ejaculate volume. But the real question is: Why would you want to? Making too much of the statistical measurements of your performance won't make sex more enjoyable. In fact, it could make it worse. "If you keep telling yourself your performance is unsatisfactory, you can wind up talking yourself into not functioning at all," says Bill Young, director of the Masters and Johnson Institute in St. Louis. "Focus on the pleasure of sex. If you're doing it to keep score, you're going to lose."

Best Test

Q. Now that I'm 50, my doctor recommends that I be screened annually for prostate cancer. He mentioned several tests, but I would like to know which is most reliable.

—*J.T., Newburyport, Massachusetts*

A. You should get two tests at your screening: a PSA blood test and a digital rectal examination. The first is a measure of a blood chemical (prostate-specific antigen) that increases if the prostate enlarges. The second, a simple physical examination of the gland, allows your doctor to feel any irregularities in its size or shape. When done together, the tests are the most effective and reliable method for detecting prostate cancer, according to William Catalona, M.D., professor and chief of the division of urologic surgery at Washington University School of Medicine in St. Louis. The annual screenings should start at age 40 if a close relative had prostate cancer.

Safe Tie Fashion

Q. Every time I buy new ties, styles change, and suddenly I'm out of date. This year all my ties are too narrow. Is there a safe width I can buy that will always be in fashion?

—*T.O., Bucksport, Maine*

A. "Safe fashion is an oxymoron," chuckles Gerald Andersen, executive director of the Neckware Association of America, a guy who has been asked this question before. Moreover, ties don't suddenly get fat or thin, which leads us to surmise that the last time you bought ties was about five years ago, when they were 2½ inches wide.

Today's ties are 3¾ inches across the base, and Anderson figures this width will be in style for at least two more years.

Fortunately, there's help for outdated neckware. Favorite old ties can easily be narrowed or widened (as long as there's enough material).

Send them to Tie Crafters, 116 East 27th Street, New York, NY 10016. They'll alter your ties and return them in two weeks.

Allergic to Condoms

Q. I think I'm allergic to latex condoms. I get a rash whenever I use one. I'm reluctant to use sheepskin condoms because I've heard they're not an effective barrier against diseases. Are there any options other than putting my sex life on hold?

—T.H., Lexington, Kentucky

A. Before you start apartment hunting in a monastery, test-drive different latex condoms. The manufacturing process differs enough from one to the next that it's possible you're just allergic to a single brand. Also, you could be reacting to the lubricant or spermicide on the condom you now use rather than to the latex itself, says Kenneth Goldberg, M.D., founder and director of the Male Health Center in Dallas. He suggests trying a nonlubricated condom.

If the rash persists, try a mild, over-the-counter steroid cream on your skin before donning the condom. You are wise to avoid using animal-skin condoms, which, as you pointed out, are not as effective a barrier against sexually transmitted diseases as latex ones are.

Avoid Wrinkles

Q. I'm 38 years old, and I'm one of those men who are trying to slow down facial wrinkling. Okay, so I'm a little vain. But tell me, does regular use of a moisturizer put the brakes on the wrinkling process? And will the use of only plain soap and water give me more wrinkles?

—W.N., Rochester, New York

A. To avoid wrinkled skin, first and foremost, stay out of the sun. Ultraviolet rays, not soap and water, are the culprits, says dermatologist Jonathan S. Weiss, M.D., a clinical assistant professor at Emory University School of Medicine.

Using moisturizers daily won't slow down the wrinkling process, but it will help disguise those crow's-feet by hydrating the skin. Dry skin, often brought on by washing with plain soap and water, makes wrinkles stand out. Switch to a moisturizing soap such as Dove or Basis for extra-dry skin, or try a soap-free cleanser such as Cetaphil.

A good defense against wrinkles, suggests Dr. Weiss, is a daily application of a fragrance-free sunscreen containing moisturizer in place of your after-shave. And if you plan to be outdoors for a long time, cover your skin with sunscreen with a sun protection factor (SPF) of at least 15.

Smoking on the Run

Q. They say balance is one of the keys to healthy living. One way I keep my balance is by allowing myself some self-indulgent activities on the weekend. One of these is a couple of cigarettes. I console myself with the promise of making up for it on my weekday morning runs. Does the increase in lung capacity I get from running help reverse the negative effects of the smoking?

—Y.H., Burlington, Vermont

A. Close, but no cigar. Although aerobic exercise can make your oxygen processing more efficient, it does little to offset the effects of smoking. Tobacco smoke, which contains more than 4,000 chemicals (43 of them known carcinogens), hinders the lungs' ability to filter out obstructions that can irritate and scar their lining. Unfortunately, exercise does little to eliminate the carcinogens or reduce the irritation caused by smoking.

About the only good news we have for you is that the hazards of smoking are usually dose-responsive: The more you smoke, the greater your risk of falling prey to smoking-related ills like lung cancer. Since you seem to be keeping your smoking to a minimum, your risk of lung disease may not be so great. But why play high-stakes poker with your health?

Vasectomy Reversal

Q. I had a vasectomy at age 31, and last year at age 34, I had it reversed. Now I have a low sperm count and my sperm has low motility, but my urologist says I still have a chance of becoming fertile again. Is there anything I can do to improve my odds?

—M.G., New York, New York

A. It depends on how low your sperm count and motility are, but the prognosis is good for men who have had a vasectomy reversed within five years, says reversal specialist Marc Goldstein, M.D., director of the Male Reproduction and Microsurgery Unit at New York Hospital–Cornell Medical Center. "In the 400 reversals I've done, 98 percent of the men who had their reversal within five years of their vasectomy regained their fertility and 75 percent managed to get their partners pregnant within two years."

Although the numbers drop a bit in men who wait up to ten years, they are still very good—95 percent and 62 percent, respectively.

Even though you still have a low sperm count and low motility, you may be fertile. Have your urologist test you to see if you have developed antisperm antibodies. Men still produce sperm after a vasectomy, but the body has to break them down internally, so it develops antibodies that attack and destroy the sperm as if it were a foreign substance. If antibodies are present, ask your urologist about treatment with prednisone or a similar steroid that suppresses the antibody response. Another option is to have your sperm "washed" with special chemicals to remove the antibodies. The "cleaned" sperm would then be injected directly into your partner's uterus when she is fertile. In vitro fertilization may also succeed, even for men with exceedingly low counts, as long as their sperm are healthy and mobile.

If none of these alternatives works, you may want to ask your urologist about having another reversal to remove any possible narrowing or leaks in your vas deferens.

Vitamin Confusion

Q. Is it a good idea to take multivitamins, or is it better to take individual supplements? My multivitamin provides 100 percent of the RDA for most vitamins and minerals, but I'm worried that taking large amounts of many nutrients every day might hurt my system. What do you think?
—*P.J., Cupertino, California*

A. Although any dietitian will tell you it is best to meet all your nutritional needs by eating a balanced diet, a standard multivitamin can be a safe and adequate supplement for athletes or people on the go. "Multivitamins are fine for you if you're not eating a wide variety of foods and feel you may be missing certain nutrients," says Martin Yadrick, a registered dietitian at the University of Kansas Medical Center.

He cautions against daily use of a multivitamin that supplies more than 100 percent of the Recommended Dietary Allowance (RDA) for many nutrients, "especially when you're talking about fat-soluble vitamins like A, D and E, which are stored in the liver and aren't easily excreted by the body."

As for individual supplements, most dietitians advise against these, since they usually supply megadoses of vitamins or minerals, which are far in excess of the RDA.

For a more specific or intense supplementation plan, check with your doctor or a registered dietitian.

Spicy Diet

Q. Does eating spicy foods like jalapeño peppers pose any health problems?

—A.R., North Hollywood, California

A. Not at all. Studies have shown that spicy foods are harmless, despite the very real feeling that they are burning the lips, mouth, throat and stomach, according to Samuel Klein, M.D., associate professor of medicine in the division of gastroenterology at the University of Texas Medical Branch. The burning sensation is caused by a chemical in the peppers (capsaicin), which tricks the nerves into signaling the brain that they are being burnt.

Spicy foods can and do cause some men heartburn. Liquid antacids made from aluminum magnesium hydroxide will put out the fire.

Lost in a Fog

Q. Although my health club has a sauna and a steam room, nobody there can tell me the particular benefits of each one. Can you defog this mystery for me?

—J.R., New York, New York

A. "There are really no therapeutic advantages or disadvantages to either one," says W. Larry Kenney, Ph.D., associate professor of applied physiology at Pennsylvania State University. Saunas rely on dry heat (up to 280°F). Steam rooms fill with, well, steam, and reach temperatures of 220°. Advocates claim that both can help stimulate weight loss, cleanse toxins from the body, clear up skin conditions and decrease recovery time after exercise.

As appealing as these claims sound, there's little physiological evidence to support them. Still, Dr. Kenney and others agree that sitting in a sauna or a steam room does *feel* good and will relax you. Doing so may be beneficial, from a psychological point of view, after a grueling workout.

Which is better, steam or sauna? "They both work equally well; it's just a matter of personal preference," says Dr. Kenney.

One word of caution: After a strenuous workout, your body temperature is already elevated, so be sure to drink plenty of fluids and cool off for 15 to 20 minutes before a sauna or steam.

Hot Hair

Q. I'm 30 years old, and every morning I blow-dry my hair before going to work. Now my hair is beginning to thin out on the top, and my wife says that I should stop blow-drying it, since this damages my hair and causes it to fall out faster. Is this true or just a lot of hot air?
—*S.A., Taos, New Mexico*

A. Although blow-drying can make hair overdry and more susceptible to splitting, it will not itself cause hair to fall out. Combing or brushing too hard, however, *can* lead to hair loss, and men frequently do brush hair vigorously while blow-drying, says Men's Health advisor John Romano, M.D., dermatologist at New York Hospital–Cornell Medical Center. He says if you blow-dry carefully and brush gently, you'll have no hair loss. First, towel-dry your hair to remove excess water. Then blow-dry, keeping the unit six to ten inches away from your hair and running it at a low to medium setting. While drying, use fingers, not a comb, to get your hair going where you want. Then *gently* style with a wide-tooth comb or brush.

Boxers or Briefs?

Q. I've heard that wearing regular briefs can make a guy sterile. If this is true, would it be better to switch to boxer shorts?
—*M.D., Sacramento, California*

A. Wearing briefs, even if they're tight fitting, will not produce any fertility problems. Just ask Jim Palmer or his two kids. Over the years researchers have theorized that briefs may interfere with a man's sperm production by holding the testicles too close to the body and thus elevating their temperature, but no studies have definitively shown this to be the case, says Jack Jaffe, M.D., medical director of the

Potency Recovery Center in Van Nuys, California. "The majority of men today wear briefs and don't have any fertility problems. But if one of my patients comes to me with fertility problems and wants to try making the switch, I tell him to go ahead. It's like eating chicken soup if you have a cold—can't hurt."

Fuzzy Kisses

Q. For years my wife has been nagging me to shave off my mustache because, she says, it feels like a broom when I kiss her. But I like it. Is there anything I can do to soften it so I stop rubbing her the wrong way?

—*S.P., San Jose, California*

A. Get a trim. "Most mustaches get in the way because they're too long," says Peter Bradley, general manager of Vidal Sassoon Salons in the United States. "It doesn't have to be big and bushy to be a problem; even a little extra can make your wife feel as if she just kissed your power sander instead of you." Also, avoid washing your mustache with regular soap. That will leave a residue that can make your mustache especially coarse. Instead, treat it like the hair on your head: Shampoo it, then rinse and apply a moisturizing conditioner. Allow the conditioner to stay on for 60 to 90 seconds and rinse again. If this doesn't make you a softie, check your local hair salon before getting out the razor; some carry special moisturizers for facial hair.

Honesty at Work

Q. Recently I was asked to gather information about a counterpart who works for one of my company's chief competitors. The method I was asked to use was at best unethical and in all likelihood illegal. When I informed my boss about my concerns, he implied that failure to do "my job" could result in being fired. What's the best way to handle the situation?

—*T.M., Cleveland, Ohio*

A. We agree with Jiminy Cricket on this one: You have to let your conscience be your guide. But listening to a lawyer wouldn't hurt, either. "What some people consider to be illegal or unethical may actually be within the boundaries of the law, so it might be wise for you to discuss your situation with someone who knows," suggests Bob Brady, publisher of *Business and Legal Reports* and an attorney who specializes in employment law. "Maybe there's a way you can do what was asked of you without having to violate your conscience.

"If you refuse to compromise your principles and are fired as a result, you could sue your employer and possibly win," adds Brady. "But you would have to prove that you were terminated because of it—and that would be difficult." It's unlikely that the reason given for your termination was that you were "too honest."

Besides the difficulty in proving your case, suing isn't a smart career move. Even if you win, once word got out that you sued your employer—and word would get out—it would be very difficult to get another job. No matter how noble your reasons, jobs don't come easy to those with a history of taking their employers to court.

In the meantime, we advise you start looking for another job—ASAP. Any boss who would fire you for your scruples would fire you for any number of lame reasons. "If you're an ethical person working for an unethical boss, the best long-term advice is to find another boss," says Brady.

Troubled Back

Q. Having had a bad back for many years, I've always been told that swimming is the best exercise for me. However, I'm not too fond of swimming and was wondering if there are any back-friendly exercises for us landlubbers.

—P.B., Endicott, New York

A. Trainers recommend swimming to anyone with a bad back because the exercise provides the double benefit of strength and aerobic conditioning without much joint and bone pounding. But swimming isn't right for everyone. "No one activity works equally well for all those with bad backs, so we usually have to experiment," says Tom Lorren, a physical therapist and director of rehabilitation at the Texas Back Institute in Dallas. He's found that choosing the right exercise depends on knowing the *kind* of back injury you have. If you have a disk problem, you might try walking, or cross-country skiing on an indoor simulator. If you have spinal stenosis (narrowing of the column that surrounds the spinal cord), your best bet is cycling or rowing. If your problem is a garden-variety muscle strain or spasm, walking or cross-country ski machines usually work best.

Before embarking on any exercise plan, have your back problem diagnosed by an orthopedist or physical therapist. Then ask him what exercise choices would be best for you.

Redneck Roughness

Q. Every time I shave, my neck gets red and a rash develops. I use a razor and a preshave lotion, but my skin still gets irritated. Is there anything I can do to minimize the damage?

—D.L., Excelsior, Minnesota

A. You're experiencing what dermatologists call pseudofolliculitis barbae. That's "razor bumps" in plain English. These bumps can take the form of a rash, or they can look like little inflamed pimples under the chin and on the neck. They're caused when sharp, newly cut whiskers curl back around and reenter the skin. Although this condition is more common among black men, others are also afflicted by it.

The easiest solution is to grow a beard, since the coiled whiskers will spring back out of the skin once they are about half an inch long. If this isn't a viable option, the tips listed below, from Oakland, California, skin-care expert Kathryn Leverette, will help you get a clean shave without the bumps.

• Soak your razor in alcohol for ten minutes before shaving.

• Use a sudsing antibacterial soap or unscented shaving cream to lather up.

• Shave only in the direction of hair growth.

• Don't stretch the skin to shave closer. When the skin bounces back, the shaved hair will be trapped below the skin line.

• After shaving, use a nonirritating, nonalcoholic tonic.

Hatless

Q. I used to wear a hat all the time, but recently stopped because several people told me that doing so would make me lose my hair. I miss my hats, but I'd miss my hair more.

—N.W., Boston, Massachusetts

A. Heredity, not headgear, determines whether a man will go bald. Wearing tight-fitting football helmets or welding masks day after day

306

can speed hair loss in men prone to baldness by decreasing the blood supply to the hair follicles, causing them to die prematurely, says Dr. John Romano. But the average hat is unlikely to pose any threat to your locks, no matter what your genetic propensity.

Fear of Speaking

Q. I dread having to speak before a crowd, yet my job demands that I occasionally give presentations to groups of up to 35 people. How can I overcome my fear and become a better speaker?

—*K.B., Walla Walla, Washington*

A. "Most of the best speakers still get a little nervous even though they've given hundreds or thousands of talks," says Al Walker, president of the National Speakers Association. "But if you're properly prepared, that nervous energy can be the difference between a flat speech and a lively one."

That being said, good speakers do use certain tricks that allow them to shine when the spotlight is on. To harness your adrenaline and improve your speaking ability, try the following:

Memorize both ends. By carefully planning an opening and a closing, you'll cut down on your prespeech anxiety, and you also won't have to spend the last third of your talk worrying about how you're going to wind things up.

Make allies. During your speech, make eye contact with various individuals in the room for a few seconds, enough to elicit a facial expression. People who acknowledge you with a smile or a nod are usually on your side, and you should turn back to them periodically throughout your speech. "Work with the people who show approval and let them win the others over," says Walker.

Have extra information. Speakers typically tend to talk much faster when they're actually giving a speech than when they are just practicing. It's a good rule of thumb to go in with twice as much information as you need so you don't run out of things to say 10 minutes into a 15-minute speech.

Practice. Consider joining a local chapter of Toastmasters International, a nonprofit organization devoted to teaching the art of public speaking. Chapter members get together weekly to take turns at the podium. Or, consider taking a public-speaking class or hiring a speech coach.

Preworkout Nibbles

Q. I've heard numerous theories on whether it's a good idea to eat before a workout. One claimed that food consumed immediately prior to a workout is not important because the energy for exercise comes from food consumed 10 to 12 hours earlier. Another stated that a small preworkout meal is essential to maximize performance. What's the best nutritional strategy to help me get the most out of my workouts?

—*M.H., Williston, Vermont*

A. Energy for exercise comes from foods eaten anytime during the 48 hours prior to exercise, *including* those consumed immediately before the workout. When deciding whether to eat before a workout, you have to consider what type of exercise you will be doing, how long it will last and when you ate your last meal, says Liz Applegate, Ph.D., author of *Power Foods*. Aerobic exercise such as running or cycling tends to last longer and burn more calories than weight workouts, and for these you may find it especially beneficial to consume a snack of 200 to 300 calories 15 to 30 minutes before starting. Ideal choices include high-carbohydrate foods like fruit, fig bars, energy bars or sports drinks. All of these can make it into the bloodstream within 15 minutes.

A snack also makes good sense before any kind of exercise if you haven't eaten for more than four hours. "To be at your best, never go into a workout without eating if you feel you have an empty stomach or are light-headed," suggests Dr. Applegate. "But avoid eating a large meal or snack because it will divert blood from working muscles into the digestive tract. Also, foods high in protein and fat are much slower to digest than carbohydrates."

For endurance workouts lasting well over an hour, it is best to eat a little before the workout and resupply at regular intervals while you exercise.

Too Few Z's

Q. As a paramedic in a large city, I'm often forced to work long hours. There are lots of nights when I get only three or four hours of sleep. Is this doing long-term damage to my body? If so, is there anything I can do to minimize the ill effects?

—*S.C., San Jose, California*

A. Getting by on three or four hours of sleep once a week won't hurt you. You may feel awful the next day, but you can probably handle it. Catch up by getting to bed earlier the next night or by grabbing a quick nap whenever you can.

If you're losing more than ten hours of sleep a week, however, you could be building up a sleep deficit that's harder to restore. According to Terry Phillips, Ph.D., D.Sc., an immunologist at George Washington University Medical Center, your immune system plummets and mental skills decline when you routinely short your body of sleep.

If that's the case, the best thing you can do is try to catch up, though doing so is not easy. Depending on the size of your sleep deficit, recovering can take a month or more. Considering the demands of your job, you may have to force yourself to go to bed earlier on those nights when you can, even if there are things you'd rather be doing. While you work on paying back your sleep debt, boost your day-to-day energy level with the following tips.

• Go for a high-protein lunch. Studies show that men whose noontime meal is high in protein have much more afternoon gusto than those who go for carbohydrates. Healthy high-protein choices include tuna, poultry and low-fat yogurt.

• Cover your bases. Take a daily multivitamin supplement to ensure that your body's getting the supplies it needs. Vitamin deficiency will only enhance your dragged-out feeling.

• Get some exercise, but not too much. A brisk ten-minute walk will increase blood circulation, sending more oxygen to the muscles and to the brain. Studies show that even brief exercise boosts energy levels for up to two hours.

Tough Tummy

Q. I've been doing a lot of stomach crunches to prepare for a physical-fitness test. In the process I've gained an inch of muscle on my stomach, and now all my pants are snug. How can I strengthen my abdominal muscles without building a "muscle potbelly"?

—*T.H., San Diego, California*

A. Although it's not impossible to gain an inch of muscle around your midsection over the course of several months, it's our guess that your new belly is made more of fat than muscle. For one thing, stomach crunches tend to isolate the upper abdominals and ignore the lower, making it very unlikely that your routine would put that much bulk around your waistline. In addition, although abdominal muscles do increase in size with use, they typically push organs inward, not out, producing a tight, washboard look, says Charles Kuntzleman, Ed.D., associate professor of physical education at the University of Michigan.

If you disagree, try the pinch-poke test. If you can pinch more than an inch of skin off your stomach or your index finger sinks into your belly past its first joint, the problem is fat, not muscle. Many men who switch from an aerobic-type fitness program to a strength- or calisthenics-based routine gain a few pounds until they adjust their diets for the fact that they're burning fewer calories, even though they're exercising just as long. To tighten your lower abdomen, Dr. Kuntzleman suggests curl-backs: Sit on the floor with your knees up and your arms crossed over your chest. Moving backward, lower your upper body until you feel a "tug." Hold for three to five seconds; return to original position. Do 10 to 15 repetitions per day.

Testy Testicles

Q. For several months I've had an ache in my testicles. Sometimes the pain is severe, sometimes mild and other times it doesn't hurt at all. I checked for any lumps that might have signaled cancer, but fortunately I didn't find any. What could be causing my pain, and is there anything I can do to make it go away?

—*E.L., Kansas City, Kansas*

A. Cancerous lumps in the testicles rarely produce any pain. (That's actually one of the reasons men need to examine themselves regularly.) Take your problem to a urologist to see if the cause might be an infection. If so, he'll probably put you on an antibiotic, which should clear up the problem in less than three weeks.

If you don't have an infection, your pain may be the result of a hernia or partially obstructed epididymis, the narrow, curly tube that coils around the outside of your testicles. Another possibility is intermittent torsion, a condition in which the testicles swivel on themselves, cutting off blood supply to the area. As the name implies, the torsion can subside only to recur; therefore, it is easier to diagnose while you're still experiencing pain. In some rare cases, testicular pain has no discernible origin. Such cases typically resolve themselves over time, but to be safe, see a doctor.

One O'Clock Shadow

Q. I've heard of a five o'clock shadow, but mine is usually visible by 1:00 P.M. I've used electric and disposable razors, but I just can't seem to get close enough to keep my whiskers down all day. What am I doing wrong?

—*D.M., West Norriton, Pennsylvania*

A. The speed of beard growth varies little, but some men like you have a very full, dark beard that makes its presence known even when it's short. The only practical thing you can do to minimize your afternoon shadow is to give yourself an ultraclose shave every morning, says Dr. John Romano. To do this without irritating your skin, start by lathering your beard with soap and warm water to soften the whiskers. Without rinsing off the soap, spread on a shaving gel, and using a sharp razor, shave in the direction of hair growth.

Keep a rechargeable electric razor in your desk drawer at work and use it for afternoon touch-ups.

Morning Eyes

Q. Many mornings when I wake up, my eyes are red and swollen. Although the problem usually clears itself up within an hour or two, it does get annoying. Is there anything I can do to see my way out of this?

—*T.C., Merritt Island, Florida*

A. Pack those bags, pal. Your problem, the result of fluid collecting around your eyes, is probably caused by sleeping on your stomach or without a pillow. This puts your head level with or below your heart and allows fluid to accumulate around your eyes. "Anytime blood has to move uphill to get back to the heart, there is an increased tendency for swelling," says ophthalmologist Thomas O. Burkholder, M.D.

The swelling dissipates when you get out of bed because gravity pulls the fluid back toward the heart. You can avoid, or minimize, that morning-zombie look by sleeping on your back or side and propping your head up with a pillow or two.

Excessive fatigue and alcohol can make the swelling worse, since they dilate the tiny vessels around the eyes and let fluid build up. If your swelling is more severe at certain times of the year, you may be suffering from allergies.

Building Trust

Q. I'm 35 and have recently begun dating a 33-year-old divorced woman who has three kids. I have a great relationship with two of her kids, but the oldest, a ten-year-old boy, won't have anything to do with me. How can I win him over?

—T.S., Lancaster, Pennsylvania

A. "Chances are, he doesn't have anything against you personally; he's just protecting his territory," says Bruce Fisher, Ed.D., author of *Rebuilding: When Your Relationship Ends*. He says that after a divorce, the oldest boy often assumes the role of the man of the family and feels he has to protect his mother from being hurt again.

To show him you're not just there to see his mother, Dr. Fisher suggests you set aside a few days a month to do something with him and his siblings. It can be a hike, a fishing trip, a baseball game or anything they enjoy. It's best if their mother doesn't come along. If she does, the boy is more likely to slip back into his role of protector.

If things don't start to improve within a few months, and you're serious about your relationship, consider some family counseling.

Index